FROM BURDENED TO BALANCED

FINDING RENEWAL THROUGH SCRIPTURE + SCIENCE

Megan Wollerton

Aurora Corialis Publishing

Pittsburgh, PA

FROM BURDENED TO BALANCED: FINDING RENEWAL THROUGH SCRIPTURE + SCIENCE
Copyright © 2025 by Megan Wollerton

All rights reserved. No part of this book may be used, reproduced, stored in a retrieval system, or transmitted by any means—electronic, mechanical, photocopy, microfilm, recording, or otherwise—without written permission from the publisher, except in the case of brief quotations embodied in critical articles or reviews. For more information, address: cori@auroracorialispublishing.com.

All external reference links utilized in this book have been validated to the best of our ability and are current as of publication. All Bible quotes are from the NIV version of the Bible, unless otherwise noted.

The publisher and the author make no guarantees concerning the level of success you may experience by following the advice and strategies contained in this book, and you accept the risk that results will differ for each individual.

Neither the authors nor the publisher assumes any responsibility for errors, omissions, or contrary interpretations of the subject matter herein. Any perceived slight of an individual or organization is purely unintentional.

To ensure privacy and confidentiality, some names or other identifying characteristics of the persons included in this book may have been changed. All the personal examples of the authors' own lives and experiences have not been altered.

Printed in the United States of America
Edited by: Allison Hrip, Aurora Corialis Publishing
Cover Design: Karen Captline, BetterBe Creative
Paperback ISBN: 978-1-958481-48-6
Ebook ISBN: 978-1-958481-49-3

Praise for *From Burdened to Balanced*

"I met Megan first as an athlete and amateur boxer and Golden Glove winner over a decade ago and watched her develop into a respected personal fitness trainer and group instructor. This book exemplifies here talents and motivation skills. I am a Christian, and the Biblical examples used in this book bring so much clarity to her reference points. The Bible brings so much wisdom to us! Megan is wise beyond her youth, and I'm looking forward to reading this book again and again!"

—Joe Divosevic, SCCC, CSCS
MAC Gym Owner/Coach

"*From Burdened to Balanced* is the book so many of us need. If you've ever felt like you're constantly pouring into others but running on empty, Megan's message will hit home. She takes self-care from something that feels selfish to something that's actually about stewardship. She helps you care for yourself so you can keep showing up for what matters!

"As someone who works with leaders juggling work, life, and faith, I see burnout all the time, and it's usually creeping in before people even notice. Megan's insights are a wake-up call and a roadmap back to balance. This book is practical, honest, and full of wisdom that sticks with you. If you're ready to get back to a place of energy and purpose, start here."

—Desiree Petrich
Bestselling Author, Keynote Speaker, and Leadership Consultant

"Megan Wollerton's book *From Burdened to Balanced* is a game-changer for anyone who looks successful but feels empty inside. Her "Four Balance Blockers" framework perfectly captures why so many high achievers end up burned out—whether it's living out of alignment with your true values, caving to others' expectations, imposing impossible standards on yourself, or chasing vague goals. I love how she shares her own journey from putting on a brave face in a toxic work environment to living authentically.

"What makes this book special is seeing how these principles have transformed not just her life but countless others she's worked with. Her practical exercises (especially that eye-opening 5-Whys technique) help you discover what truly matters beneath surface-level goals. I've witnessed firsthand how her faith-centered, values-driven approach has allowed her to lift herself up and now lift others in such an authentic way. If you're successful but feeling stuck or lost, her blend of spiritual wisdom and practical steps offers exactly the replenishment you're looking for."

—Christie Cawley
People & Culture Executive | Leadership Coach | Community Wellness Advocate

"In her new book, *From Burdened to Balanced*, Megan masterfully blends scientific research with biblical wisdom to highlight the significance of self-care in today's fast-paced world. Drawing on psychology, neuroscience, and wellness studies, this book emphasizes the vital connection between physical, mental, and emotional well-being.

"From my own experience of juggling so many hats, I can truly attest to this. From being a mama of five, a wife, an ordained minister, a published author, a board-certified youth mental health coach, and a high-impact tutor for elementary students nationwide to being an independent holistic/proactive wellness distributor for Three International, I understand how crucial self-care really is. What sets this book apart is its seamless integration of scripture, illustrating how God's Word supports the practice of self-care. Passages from the Bible are woven throughout, reminding us that nurturing our minds, seeking peace, and honoring our bodies—the temple of the Holy Spirit— are all essential to living out God's purpose for our lives.

"This thought-provoking work encourages readers to embrace self-care not as selfishness but as a biblical command to steward our bodies and souls. Whether you are seeking practical advice or spiritual guidance, this book provides a refreshing perspective on why self-care is not only important for health but also essential for fulfilling God's calling. It is a powerful reminder that caring for oneself is part of caring for God's creation."

—Judi Logan,
Minister, Author, Speaker, and Business Owner

"I love this book. No matter where you are in your self-care journey, reading it will infuse you with high vibes to lovingly set boundaries, establish a plan for self-care, and prioritize it rather than happening to experience it or practice it when life allows—which is usually never! There is so much wisdom and love and light within each page. I highly recommend it!"

—Marta Sauret Greca
Speaker, Coach, and Bestselling Author

"*From Burdened to Balanced* is a transformative guide that speaks directly to the heart of every Christian who has ever felt overwhelmed by the weight of serving. With wisdom, vulnerability, reflective questions, and deep biblical insight, Megan reminds us that self-care is not selfish—it is stewardship. Her personal journey from burnout to balance is both relatable and inspiring, offering practical steps rooted in scripture and science to help readers realign with God's purpose. This book is a must-read for anyone seeking renewal, restoration, and a healthier way to serve both God and others."

—Dr. Christina Fontana
Transformational Business Coach + Professional Speaker

"Megan Wollerton understands the intersection of faith, wellness, and mental resilience like few others. *From Burdened to Balanced* is an essential guide for anyone seeking a biblical and practical approach to avoiding burnout and embracing true balance. She shares actionable strategies deeply rooted in faith principles. This book will help you make sustainable changes that honor both your calling and your well-being. I highly recommend it!"

—David McGlennen
Fractional CEO and Executive Coach

"*From Burdened to Balanced* is the reset button we all need—whether you're launching your career, navigating the messy middle, or approaching life's next chapter. It's a guide, not just for reflection, but for action. It challenges you to stop settling—in work, in life, and in the expectations you place on yourself—and to finally define what success and alignment truly mean for you. It's never too late (or too early) to pause, reassess, and reclaim balance—mentally, socially, spiritually, and professionally. This book reminds us that we're not alone on this journey, and that by taking care of ourselves, we become better for those around us. More than a book—it's a personal call to action."

—Cambria W. Zebley
Crumbl Franchise Owner, Operator

"Too busy for another self-help book? That's exactly why you need this one! *From Burdened to Balanced* isn't here to add to your to-do list—it's here to strip away the noise and force you to take a hard look at where you are and why you keep settling for imbalance. Whether you're climbing the ladder, stuck in neutral, or figuring out your next move, this book calls BS on the excuses we all make and helps you get real about what success actually looks like—mentally, socially, spiritually, and professionally. It's part gut check, part guide, and all about owning your story before someone else writes it for you."
—Pete Schramm
Founder, CEO, Author, Speaker

Table of Contents

Introduction: How We Got Here i

Chapter One The Four Balance Blockers 1

Chapter Two Purpose/Existential Wellness 11

Chapter Three Mental Wellness 25

Chapter Four Emotional Wellness 37

Chapter Five Physical Wellness 51

Chapter Six Environmental Wellness 65

Chapter Seven Relational Wellness 75

Chapter Eight Financial Wellness 89

Conclusion 101

Introduction: How We Got Here

In the Christian community, serving is what we do. We learn that we are the body of Christ, His hands and feet. I see so many of my brothers and sisters in Christ pouring their hearts into ministry, volunteering, and trying to do it all. But honestly, a lot of them are overburdened and burning out. I've watched as they continue to show up and check the boxes, but you can tell they're running on empty. They're exhausted and resentful, but they keep going because they think that if they step back, say no to a project, or even pause to practice a little self-care, it's selfish or wrong. The truth is that Scripture tells us something completely different. God does not want us to be burdened; He calls us to take care of ourselves. Self-care is not an act of selfishness but an act of stewardship. Our bodies, minds, and spirits are gifts from Him, and taking care of them helps us serve Him and others better.

I'll never forget a time when I was completely stretched to the limit. Between work, family, and all my commitments, I was running on fumes spiritually, emotionally, mentally, and physically. I worked in the oil and gas industry during the Marcellus Shale boom in Pennsylvania. As a service director, I was on call all the time and worked 60-100 hours a week. Early in my career, I received a call from a drill site manager, and he said something to me I never forgot. In his thick Texan accent, he said, "Miss Megan, my drill rig runs twenty-four hours a day, seven days a week. Each day you don't keep my rig running, you're costing us about a million dollars a day. So, if you want to be successful in your job, you better be on call twenty-four seven."

At the time, I was in my twenties, full of energy, and thought I could handle it. But the nonstop demands took a serious toll. I became distant from my husband, my only friends were my coworkers, and I started relying on alcohol to deal with the stress and loneliness that I felt. Then, out of nowhere, I was let go from my job. My employer made me sign a one-year non-compete agreement, which meant I couldn't get another job in my field. The severance package they offered gave me financial stability, so I decided to take the time to focus on myself.

I wasn't unemployed for two weeks before I started to realize just how burned out I really was. I spent time reflecting, got more involved in my church, and reached out to friends. I learned something important: self-care isn't selfish, and it isn't about escaping your responsibilities; it's about realigning with God's purpose and finding renewal in His presence. That is when I decided I would not return to the oil and gas industry; I wanted to help people like me—those who put themselves on the back burner while serving others or climbing the corporate ladder.

This is what inspired me to achieve several certifications in health, fitness, nutrition, psychology, and more. It is also what motivated me to start an organization focused on helping others who are experiencing the same burnout I went through. Once I had developed my programs, I knew I wanted to write a book about life balance and self-care. However, I was torn about how to approach it. When I spoke to some business partners about my idea for this book, I heard things like, "Coming out as a Christian can be costly for your business." They reminded me of examples of other businesses that stood on their Christian values: cake bakers, website designers, and coaches who proclaimed their faith and were quickly attacked for their stances.

I was advised to write my business book first and then work on a book like this one later. That's when all progress on my book came to a halt. I tried to work on the book for three years, but I got no further than the introduction and a few paragraphs. In March of 2024, I attended a women's retreat with my church. We studied John 15:1-17, the verses about *The Vine and the Branches*. The theme for the retreat was *Abide*. On the first evening, we read the passage together. Then, we were asked to read it again, reflect on what stood out, and read it a third time, focusing on the part that resonated most.

I was immediately drawn to verse five, "Apart from me, you can do nothing." It hit me hard. I realized that when I had taken God out of the equation, I made no progress on this book or any other new project I had tried to start. I was stuck. That retreat reignited something in me. I came home, and the first thing I did was work on this book.

This book is a journey into scriptural self-care. Together, we'll explore what it means to care for ourselves as God intended, grounding our practices in biblical wisdom and practical strategies. Whether you're feeling overwhelmed or simply seeking a deeper connection with God, this is your invitation to find balance, renewal, and peace through His Word.

Before diving into self-care, I want to take a moment to ensure you are ready to embark on this journey. You need to understand that loving yourself and caring for yourself is not selfish; it's scriptural. If you are a follower of Jesus, you most likely know, from Matthew 22:36-40, that Jesus is asked which is the greatest commandment in the law. "Jesus replied: 'Love the Lord your God with all your heart and with all your soul and with all your mind.' This is the first and greatest commandment. And the second is like it: *'Love your neighbor as yourself.'* All the Law and the Prophets hang on these two commandments" (NIV, emphasis mine). This is what prompted the story of the good Samaritan.

If you grew up in a church like me, you could probably recite this verse word for word. As a kid in vacation Bible school, I memorized it. The law Jesus speaks of comes from Leviticus 19:18, "'Do not seek revenge or bear a grudge against anyone among your people, but love your neighbor as yourself. I am the LORD.'" The Lord commands us to *love our neighbors as ourselves*. Many Christians use this scripture to fuel their missions and volunteer efforts. But embedded in this directive is a profound yet often truth: we must first love ourselves. Without a healthy sense of self-love, our ability to truly extend love and care to others is limited.

Many of us focus on the first part of that verse, loving others, without fully understanding how to love ourselves. Taking the time to love ourselves isn't selfish or indulgent; it's foundational. When we prioritize our physical, emotional, mental, and spiritual well-being, we equip ourselves to live out this biblical principle in its fullest form. By cultivating balance and renewal in our lives, we can reflect on a more profound, authentic love for those around us.

I coach clients from a deep health perspective, focusing on seven areas of wellness: Purpose/Existential, Mental, Emotional, Physical, Environmental, Relational, and Financial. Each of these areas plays a crucial role in overall well-being, and this book is designed to help you explore them in depth. Every chapter is filled with scientific research and scripture to offer a fresh perspective on what it truly means to find balance and practice self-care. You'll also find practical habits and actionable steps to help you strengthen each area and incorporate self-care into your daily life.

But before we dive into these seven areas, it's important to address the setbacks that can stand in your way—what I call The Four Balance Blockers. These mindset traps can throw you off course, making it harder to maintain balance and sustain well-being. Understanding them will help you navigate challenges and create lasting change as you move through this journey.

As you work through this book, I encourage you to take your time and reflect on what you learn. Think about how you can apply these ideas to your own life to practice self-care and find a better life balance. If you want additional support or resources, a free guide accompanying this book is available at www.burdenedtobalancedbook.com.

Remember, this journey isn't about perfection; it's about progress. As you explore these concepts, I hope you find the encouragement and tools to align with God's purpose for your life, fostering a deeper connection with Him and the people He's called you to serve.

Chapter One
The Four Balance Blockers

Over the past several years, I've worked with clients struggling with burnout while chasing a wide range of goals. Some wanted to lose weight, others aimed to build strength or improve athletic performance, and many were simply trying to survive the relentless demands of daily life. No matter what their specific goal was, I kept noticing the same patterns.

As I reflected on these trends, I identified what I now call The Four Balance Blockers, or four mindset traps that throw us off balance in life. When we feel misaligned or on the brink of burnout, it's usually because one (or more) of these mental barriers is at play. These roadblocks were the most common challenges my clients faced, and learning how to overcome them unlocked their success.

It's important to keep these Balance Blockers in mind as you continue reading. Sometimes, simply naming these mental traps makes it easier to recognize them in your own life. As you go through this book, pay attention to areas where you struggle and refer back to these traps to identify which one you tend to fall into. Once you pinpoint the patterns holding you back, you can start developing a plan to overcome them and achieve better balance in your life.

The first Balance Blocker is Incongruence (a mindset trap), which occurs when a person's beliefs and actions are not aligned. For example, a client might say, "I wish I had more time to spend with my friends." Yet, when those same friends call and invite them out, the client makes excuses to stay home, choosing instead to binge-watch Netflix. Their stated desire to spend more time with friends doesn't match their actual behavior of staying home alone.

This misalignment can stem from various underlying issues. For instance, it could be a form of imposter syndrome, where the person feels unworthy of the luxury of socializing. Alternatively, they may not feel a sense of belonging within the friend group. As researcher Brené Brown has found, the opposite of belonging is fitting in.[i] If my client felt they were merely trying to fit in, the effort to maintain that facade might feel exhausting, leading them to retreat rather than engage.

When we hide behind a facade, we lose the ability to connect with others and drift further away from our true selves. This feeling of disconnection can be particularly common during significant life transitions, such as having a new child or experiencing a midlife crisis. During these times, external pressures like family issues, financial concerns, or health challenges can cause us to lose sight of what truly matters. Our relationships with loved ones may suffer, leaving us feeling exhausted and isolated. Over time, this disconnection from our authentic selves can lead to depression, stress, and a profound sense of fear or isolation.

I experienced this firsthand while working in the oil and gas industry. As a service manager for a company that provided trucking and housing for rig hands, engineers, and drill site managers, I often felt inadequate. My role required me to manage emergencies, organize crews, and oversee on-site operations with authority. I spoke with confidence, led my teams effectively, and handled harassment attempts with grace, but beneath the surface, I constantly questioned whether I was doing enough.

The facade I was trying to maintain, coupled with the anxiety of making a mistake, weighed heavily on me, dominating my thoughts and eroding my confidence. Unfortunately, the culture within the company only amplified this fear. The owner viewed every failure not as an honest mistake but as a deliberate act of incompetence or laziness. This mindset created a toxic environment where employees, including myself, were too afraid to take risks, admit errors, or even ask for help. We lived in constant fear of harsh judgment or punishment.

To overcome incongruence, we must take a step back and honestly evaluate our lives. Are we living in alignment with our values and beliefs? By reconnecting with our authentic selves, we can find balance, move toward congruence, and create a life that feels both purposeful and fulfilling.

This is exactly what I did when I left the oil and gas industry. I took time to reflect on what I truly valued and what mattered most to me. I vowed never to hide my authentic self again, no matter the circumstances. As Luke 12:2 reminds us, "There is nothing concealed that will not be disclosed, or hidden that will not be made known." The truth will always come to light, so let's live transparently before God and others. Authenticity shines brightest when we act with honesty and integrity, aligning our actions with who we truly are.

Take time to reflect on what truly matters to you. What do you value above all else? Identify three or four key values or goals that are most important in your life. Once you've clarified those, you can shape your days and decisions around them.

For example, my top values include building my relationship with my Lord and Savior, strengthening my bond with my husband and children, and growing my business by helping others achieve balance in their lives. When an opportunity arises, like traveling across the country with a friend to hear a speaker I admire, I use my values to guide my decision-making. I ask myself:

- Will this build my relationship with God?
- Will this strengthen my connection with my family?
- Will this help me grow my business in a meaningful way to serve more people?

If the answer is *no* to all questions, I know it's not the right choice for me.

By framing my decisions through the lens of my values, I can set healthy boundaries and stay true to my beliefs. This process helps me take purposeful action on what aligns with my goals and release what doesn't serve me. In doing so, I manage my time and energy more effectively, creating space to grow into a more authentic version of myself.

The second Balance Blocker is External Stigma, which refers to the pressure to meet the expectations of others. It's the belief that you must do something because someone else expects it of you. For example, you might feel compelled to get into a prestigious college because it's what your mother wants, perform exceptionally at work because it's what your boss demands, or fit into a size-two pair of jeans because society promotes that ideal.

External stigmas lead to people pleasing; this is when we allow others to dictate our lives. Much like incongruence, people pleasing or living under external stigmas prevents us from being authentic. However, while incongruence often stems from a subconscious disconnect between our beliefs and actions, external stigmas are usually clear and conscious. We know we're trying to please others, whether it's out of a fear of disappointing them or a desire to be accepted.

External stigmas prevent us from living authentically, creating unnecessary stress and imbalance. Recognizing and addressing these pressures is essential to regain control of one's life.

Start by clarifying your values. Once you have a clear understanding of what truly matters to you, reflect on the sources of external stigma in your life. Identify the external expectations you feel most pressured to meet. Ask yourself:

- Whose approval am I seeking?
- What expectations am I trying to fulfill?
- Why is it important that I meet expectations?

For example, are you chasing career success to impress your boss, or are you dieting to conform to societal beauty standards? Pinpointing the origin of these pressures is the first step toward overcoming them.

Next, focus on setting healthy boundaries. Learn to say no to activities or requests that don't align with your values and goals. Clearly and assertively communicate your boundaries without guilt. For instance, you might politely decline extra responsibilities at work if they don't support your priorities or step away from conversations that perpetuate unhealthy societal norms.

The key to addressing pressure from others is to communicate openly with those in your life who expect you to be someone you are not. Many clients struggle with this stigma for fear of upsetting another person. However, it is not selfish to prioritize your own needs from time to time, and standing up for your values is essential.

- **Galatians 1:10**, "Am I now trying to win the approval of human beings, or of God? Or am I trying to *please people*? If I were still trying to *please people*, I would not be a servant of Christ" (emphasis mine).
- **Romans 12:2**, "Do not conform to the pattern of this world but be transformed by the renewing of your mind. Then you will be able to test and approve what God's will is—his good, pleasing and perfect will."

We are not called to conform to the expectations of others but to stay true to who we are. Each of us is uniquely and wonderfully made. When you understand your gifts and values, you gain the ability to set healthy boundaries, freeing yourself from external pressures. This allows you to live a more balanced and authentic life.

The third Balance Blocker is Internal Stigma, the belief that you must do or be something specific to avoid feeling like a failure. For example, you might feel the need to bake homemade cookies for your child's school bake sale instead of simply buying premade ones. Realistically, no one at the school would mind if you brought store-bought cookies; they'd just be glad to have something to sell. But internally, you'd feel like a failure or a bad parent if you didn't create the perfect homemade cookies.

Internal stigmas push us to live up to impossible standards that no one else is imposing on us. Even when people around you say things like, "Why are you trying so hard?" or "No one expects you to be perfect," you might dismiss their words as insincere. Deep down, you tell yourself the harsh truth: *I'm just not good enough.*

This relentless self-criticism can be exhausting and isolating, making it difficult to find balance and embrace your true worth. Recognizing and challenging these internal stigmas is essential to breaking free from their hold.

The first step toward overcoming this stigma is to recognize it. Internal stigma is often the hardest to identify out of all the mindset traps. Many of my clients have internalized an *I'm not good enough* mentality and accepted it as an unchangeable truth. To start acknowledging the unrealistic expectations you place on yourself, ask: *Would I hold someone else to this same standard?* Often, the answer is no. Understanding that these pressures are self-imposed is the first step toward overcoming them.

The next step is to challenge the idea of perfectionism. Many of us fall into an *all-or-nothing* mindset. This is especially common with clients trying to lose weight. For instance, if they slip up and order pizza for lunch, they might think their entire diet is ruined and decide to indulge in a soda and cookie as well. How often have you started a diet, made a mistake, and thought, *Oh well, I'll just try again tomorrow?* Instead of striving for perfection, focus on progress. Remind yourself that something is better than nothing and that done is better than perfect. For example, store-bought cookies still fulfill the need in the bake sale example and allow you to spend your time and energy on other priorities.

Finally, practice self-compassion. Speak to yourself with the same kindness you would show a close friend. Use affirmations such as *I am enough as I am*, or *My worth is not tied to how much I achieve*. Many clients find comfort and strength in using Bible verses as part of their affirmation practice to overcome this stigma. Here are three of the most popular ones they turn to:

1. **Psalm 139:14**, "I praise you because I am fearfully and wonderfully made; your works are wonderful, I know that full well."

    Affirmation: *I am fearfully and wonderfully made by God.*

2. **Philippians 4:13**, "I can do all this through him who gives me strength."

    Affirmation: *I am capable of all things through Christ's strength.*

3. **1 Peter 2:9**, "But you are a chosen people, a royal priesthood, a holy nation, God's special possession, that you may declare the praises of him who called you out of darkness into his wonderful light."

    Affirmation: *I am chosen, holy, and God's treasured possession.*

The final barrier to balance is ambiguity; this is one of the most common issues I see in my daily work with clients. It's also the easiest to overcome when appropriately addressed. Ambiguity arises when you lack a clear objective or a defined measure of success. Without clarity, you'll find yourself spinning your wheels, quickly leading to overwhelm, feelings of failure, and eventually burnout.

When you lack a clear objective or a defined measure of success, how do you know when you've achieved your goal? Many of my clients come to me with broad statements like, "I want to be successful," "I want to be a good parent," or "I want to be healthy." While these are admirable aspirations, the first step is to define what these goals actually mean. What does success look like to you? What makes someone a good parent? What does "healthy" feel like in your life?

Setting SMART: Specific, Measurable, Achievable, Relevant, and Time-bound goals is a great starting point, but it's not enough. You need to dig deeper to uncover the driving force behind your goals. Why do you want to achieve these goals? What makes them so important to you? Understanding your "why" provides the motivation to keep pushing forward, even when times get tough.

This is where the 5-Whys practice from the certification course, Essentials of Nutrition and Coaching, comes in.[ii] I use this exercise with all my coaching clients to identify the deeper purpose behind their goals, and it's simple enough to do on your own. The process involves asking yourself *why* at least five times to drill down to the root of your motivation. Here's an example:

Client's Goal: "I want to lose twenty pounds."

Why 1: Why do you want to lose twenty pounds specifically?

Client: "Because ten years ago, I was twenty pounds lighter, and I felt better, and I had more energy."

Why 2: Why is feeling better and having more energy important to you now?

Client: "Because I'm expecting grandbabies soon, and I want to enjoy time with them and help my daughter."

Why 3: Why is helping your daughter and keeping up with your grandbabies a goal for you?

Client: "Because I worked so much when my kids were little, I feel like I missed out on quality time with them. I want to make up for that lost time."

Why 4: Why is quality time and making up for past neglect important to you?

Client: "Because I don't want to have regrets or drift apart from my family as I get older."

Why 5: Why is drifting apart from your family a problem for you?

Client: "Because I want strong relationships with my family as I age. I don't want to end up alone."

Through this exercise, it becomes clear that the client's real goal isn't simply to lose twenty pounds. Her sincere desire is to build strong, healthy relationships with her family so she can have a supportive network as she grows older. Weight loss is just a means to that end; it's not the ultimate objective. Her real goal is to create a life where she doesn't feel alone in her later years. By using the 5-Whys practice, you can uncover the deeper motivations behind your goals. Download our 5-Whys worksheet at www.burdenedtobalancedbook.com.

Using this knowledge, you can set SMART goals with a clear purpose. Drawing a line in the sand and knowing when you've accomplished your goal is key. For the client in our earlier example, a SMART goal might be babysitting her grandchildren two days a week to help her daughter work or run errands. Combining the 5-Whys exercise with SMART goal setting allows you to focus on what truly matters and creates meaningful, purpose-driven objectives.

Most importantly, when it comes to overcoming ambiguity, you must celebrate your successes. Many goal-oriented individuals tend to jump from one goal to the next, constantly pushing themselves to achieve more. While striving for growth is admirable, burnout often creeps in when we fail to pause and acknowledge our accomplishments.

When you reach a goal or achieve a milestone, take time to reflect on *how* you succeeded and celebrate it. Too often, clients who feel burned out end their days focusing on the unfinished items on their to-do lists. They go to bed thinking about what they didn't accomplish, which fuels negative self-talk and stress.

To counter this, I recommend a simple exercise: write down three things that went well during your day before going to sleep. These could be small tasks, like emptying the dishwasher, or significant achievements, like closing a business deal. Celebrating even the smallest wins helps shift your mindset, builds positivity, and reinforces your progress.

As you continue reading this book and exploring each area of deep health, keep the Four Balance Blockers in mind: Incongruence, External Stigmas, Internal Stigmas, and Ambiguity. Take time to identify which of these may be holding you back as you develop your plan to enhance your well-being and create greater balance in your life. Each chapter offers practical ideas to help you incorporate more self-care strategies, so don't let these mindset traps stand in the way of achieving your wellness goals.

Chapter Two
Purpose/Existential Wellness

Before diving into the areas of health you may be more familiar with, it's important to first examine your purpose, or what some might call existential health. When discussing this wellness dimension, many people immediately associate it with religion or faith. Questions about beliefs, the meaning of life, and spirituality often arise.

However, not everyone identifies with a particular faith. I've worked with many clients who are atheists, agnostics, or uncertain about their beliefs. If that resonates with you, I like to describe this area of wellness simply as your *reason for being*.

What gets you out of bed in the morning? What drives you to succeed, work hard, or pursue your goals? What gives your life meaning? Without a sense of purpose, it can be easy to feel aimless or unmotivated—like life is just passing by.

The Japanese culture offers a beautiful concept called *ikigai*. The word *ikigai* combines *iki* (life) and *gai* (reason or worth). It's based on the idea that finding a personalized sense of purpose can lead to a more fulfilling and meaningful life. *Ikigai* has caught a lot of attention over the last few years, and even the National Institutes of Health (NIH) studied if having a purpose in life enhances health and well-being and if the broader Japanese concept of *ikigai* may similarly contribute to positive physical and psychosocial outcomes.

The NIH conducted a nationwide longitudinal study of Japanese adults aged sixty-five and older and examined the impact of *ikigai* on various health and well-being outcomes over three years. Participants with *ikigai* experienced significant benefits, including a 31 percent lower risk of developing functional disability and a 36 percent lower risk of dementia.[iii] They also reported fewer depressive symptoms, greater happiness, higher life satisfaction, and increased participation in social activities such as hobby clubs. These effects were particularly pronounced among men. The findings suggest that *ikigai* plays a crucial role in promoting physical, psychological, and social well-being in older adults.

This is not just for the benefit of older adults, though. In another study, 43,391 Japanese adults explored the relationship between *ikigai* (a sense of life worth living) and cause-specific mortality risk. Over seven years, participants who reported not having ikigai faced a 50 percent higher risk of all-cause mortality compared to those who did. The absence of *ikigai* was significantly linked to increased mortality from cardiovascular disease (60 percent higher risk) and external causes (90 percent higher risk) but not from cancer.[iv] These findings highlight the vital role of *ikigai* in reducing mortality risks, particularly related to heart health and external factors, emphasizing the importance of a meaningful sense of purpose in life.

Ikigai is a concept that's gaining traction, especially among millennials like me, who crave more purpose in our work. I remember a time when I was trying to choose a college path and discussing my interests with my parents. I was met with responses like, "You don't want to do that; there's no money in it." Like many of my peers, I was steered toward practical careers—things that paid well and were in demand—but not necessarily things I was passionate about.

That's how I initially landed in the oil and gas industry. I had just graduated from college, and the industry was booming— right at the start of the Marcellus Shale expansion and the rise of fracking in Pennsylvania. There was money to be made and plenty of job openings, but I had no background in the industry. I knew nothing about oversized load hauling, trucking logistics, drill site safety, or operations. More importantly, I had no passion for it; I simply didn't care. Missing two of the four key elements of *ikigai* (passion and skill) is what set me on the path to burnout.

Over time, I developed the skills and became very good at my job, but my heart was never in it. And that's the key: finding your *ikigai* isn't just about being good at something or making money; it's about aligning your work with what truly fulfills you. Without that alignment, burnout is almost inevitable.

To discover your *ikigai,* you need to reflect on four key questions. The intersection of your answers forms your unique purpose. Below, I've outlined these questions, and a Venn diagram-style exercise can be downloaded for free from this book's resource page at www.burdenedtobalancedbook.com.

1. **What do you love?**
   What are the things you genuinely enjoy? Maybe you love writing, painting, building things, or solving complex problems. Our culture often suggests that what we love should remain hobbies, but *ikigai* challenges this notion by tying it to our greater purpose.

2. **What are you good at?**
   What skills or talents do you possess? Are you good at math, science, building computers, or do you have unique physical abilities? While society may say that being good at something doesn't mean you should pursue it, *ikigai* encourages alignment between your talents and purpose.

3. **What can you be paid for?**
   What skills or services can you offer that others would pay you to do? This question bridges the gap between passion and practicality, helping you identify ways to sustain your purpose financially.

4. **What does the world need?**
   Where do you see opportunities to make an impact? Is there a need in your community or the world that aligns with your skills and passions?

Reflecting on these questions helps create a clearer picture of your *ikigai*. By finding the overlap between these areas, you can uncover your purpose and live with greater intention and fulfillment. While the Bible doesn't explicitly mention *ikigai*, its principles of finding purpose, using God-given gifts, and living a meaningful life align beautifully with many biblical teachings. Here are some examples of how *ikigai* can be supported by scripture.

What do you love?

The Bible emphasizes the importance of finding joy in God and the gifts He provides. From a biblical perspective, the things we love often reflect the desires that God has placed in our hearts. When we delight in the Lord and align our passions with His will, He shapes those desires into a meaningful purpose.

Each of us is drawn to different things in this world. The diversity in art, for example, arises from our unique perspectives on beauty. It is essential to embrace this individuality as we consider our purpose and set our goals.

Psalm 37:4 states, "Delight yourself in the Lord, and He will give you the desires of your heart" (ESV). This verse reminds us that by pursuing what we love in harmony with God's guidance, we can experience both fulfillment and spiritual growth.

In Colossians 3:23, we see how we are to work with all our hearts. "Whatever you do, work at it with all your heart, as working for the Lord, not for human masters." Paul reminds us that our work, whatever it may be, should be done with enthusiasm and passion as if we are serving God directly. This means that even our smallest efforts can honor Him when done wholeheartedly and with the right attitude.

You find your mission in the *ikigai* model, where *what you love* overlaps with *what the world needs*. Your mission is something you do out of passion and necessity, but it lacks the elements of *what you're good at* and *what you can be paid for*. This often means volunteer work or service-driven efforts.

When you're operating in your mission, you may not be the best at it, and you probably aren't making much money from it, but it's something the world needs, and you feel called to provide it. If you find yourself in this space, you have two of the four circles of *ikigai* overlapping. Think about volunteer work you've done or missionaries you've heard of—people who feel led to serve in meaningful ways despite the challenges. God may place incredible opportunities on your heart to help those in need, but it's important to remember that while mission is a powerful part of your journey, it is not the complete picture of *ikigai*. It is not your purpose.

What are you good at?

Now, where what you are good at and what you love overlap, you get your passion. When you love doing something, you will get a hit of dopamine in your brain—that feel-good chemical—and this will lead you to repeat that behavior and become good at it. I believe God wires us this way to prepare us for our purpose. He helps us develop the skills so that when we align with his plan for our life, we will have both the love and the skills needed to fulfill what is required.

The Bible frequently discusses using our God-given talents and abilities for His glory and the benefit of others. Each of us has unique gifts meant to be shared. Our abilities are gifts from God, entrusted to us as stewards. As Peter reminds us, every good thing we have comes from God and is meant to be used to serve others. Viewing our talents as opportunities for service allows us to fulfill our purpose as God's set apart people. This is seen in 1 Peter 4:10, "Each of you should use whatever gift you have received to serve others, as faithful stewards of God's grace in its various forms." Our talents are not simply ours to keep; they are entrusted to us by God to serve others and fulfill His purpose for our lives.

In 1 Corinthians 12:8-10, Paul explains that God intentionally and uniquely gives us our abilities and gifts through the Holy Spirit. Each believer receives different gifts, not earned, chosen, or self-generated, but lovingly distributed by the Spirit according to God's perfect plan. These gifts reflect His creativity and desire for us to work together in unity, each playing a distinct and vital role in His kingdom.

Paul highlights that this diversity in gifts is by design. No one has every gift, and no gift is more important than another. This is a beautiful reminder that our differences are meant to complement one another, creating a unified body where every part has a purpose. Just as a physical body relies on the unique functions of each organ to thrive, so too does the body of Christ rely on its members' varied talents and abilities.

1 Corinthians 12:8-11 states:

> To one there is given through the Spirit a message of wisdom, to another a message of knowledge by means of the same Spirit, to another faith by the same Spirit, to another gifts of healing by that one Spirit, to another miraculous powers, to another prophecy, to another distinguishing between spirits, to another speaking in different kinds of tongues, and to still another the interpretation of tongues. All these are the work of one and the same Spirit, and he distributes them to each one, just as he determines.

This teaches us that no matter how differently we are gifted or abled, each talent holds equal value and purpose in God's plan. Our gifts are not meant to glorify ourselves or set us apart as superior but to reflect God's glory and serve others. Whether it is the ability to lead, teach, encourage, or offer acts of mercy, every gift is critical in building up the community of believers and sharing God's love with the world.

By using our gifts to serve others, we step into the unique role God has designed for each of us. This not only fulfills our personal purpose but also strengthens the unity and effectiveness of the larger community. Through the faithful stewardship of our God-given talents, we bring honor to Him and embody His love and grace in tangible ways.

What can you be paid for?

If you use your talents and gifts solely to make money, according to the *ikigai* concept, that is considered a profession, not your purpose. It leaves out what you love and what the world may need, focusing only on what you are good at and what you can be paid for. In today's world, where so much emphasis is placed on material success and keeping up with societal standards, we often sacrifice our passions and higher calling in the pursuit of wealth. This imbalance can lead to stress and burnout.

It's important to note that there is nothing wrong with being wealthy. We'll explore this further in the Financial Wellness chapter. Scripture affirms the dignity of honest work and the value of earning a living. When we work with integrity and purpose, we honor God while providing for ourselves and others.

However, true *ikigai* requires all four elements to be in harmony: what you love, what you are good at, what you can be paid for, and what the world needs. Leaving any one of these out means you're not fully living out your purpose. Achieving balance among these elements not only brings fulfillment but also aligns your work with a higher calling.

Several passages of scripture discuss getting paid wages: Leviticus 19:13, "'Do not defraud or rob your neighbor. Do not hold back the wages of a hired worker overnight,'" and Deuteronomy 24:14-15, "Do not take advantage of a hired worker who is poor and needy, whether that worker is a fellow Israelite or a foreigner residing in one of your towns. Pay them their wages each day before sunset, because they are poor and are counting on it. Otherwise they may cry to the LORD against you, and you will be guilty of sin."

Scripture affirms the dignity of honest work and the value of earning a living. When we work with integrity and purpose, we honor God and provide for ourselves and others.

What does the world need?

Just look around, there are so many gaps that need filling. We do not live in a perfect world; there are always people to help and problems to solve. What do you see around you that the world needs? The Bible calls us to serve others and meet the needs of the world around us. Purpose often arises from identifying where we can bring light, love, and hope to others. If you are a follower of Jesus, then you know we are to serve others as it was written in Mark 10:45, "For even the Son of Man did not come to be served, but to serve, and to give his life as a ransom for many."

Jesus's teachings emphasize that we are called to serve others, which aligns beautifully with the *ikigai* principle of fulfilling what the world needs. In Mark 10:43–44, Jesus says that true greatness comes from becoming a servant to others. This servanthood reflects the deeper purpose we are designed for: to meet the needs of those around us in alignment with God's will.

Jesus Himself modeled this through His life as the Suffering Servant (Isaiah 53:11). While his ultimate service was to God, He demonstrated what it means to act selflessly for the benefit of others. In the same way, we are called to step into roles where we meet the needs of the powerless, the marginalized, and the broken.

There can always be too much of a good thing. Taking anything to an extreme, no matter how noble, becomes unhealthy. Serving others is an important part of our human experience, but we have to recognize that we *cannot* pour from an empty cup. The purpose of this book is to help prevent burnout and overwhelm, and part of that means understanding the balance between giving and restoring ourselves.

We've already discussed the dangers of external stigmas and people-pleasing, and even Jesus himself modeled the importance of rest. He didn't grind himself into exhaustion just for the sake of doing more—he knew when to step away and recharge. Throughout scripture, we see Jesus intentionally withdrawing to find solitude. After hearing of John the Baptist's death in Matthew 14:13, "he withdrew by boat privately to a solitary place." In Mark 6:45-46, he sent his disciples ahead by boat while he stayed behind, retreating to a mountain to pray. These moments weren't acts of avoidance; they were acts of renewal.

If Jesus, who carried the weight of the world's salvation, took time to rest, why do we feel guilty for doing the same? Rest isn't a luxury; it's a necessity. It allows us to show up fully, serve others effectively, and sustain our purpose without losing ourselves in the process.

But rest isn't about stepping away from our purpose, it's what allows us to fulfill it. The concept of *ikigai* teaches that our purpose is incomplete without addressing what the world needs. For Christians, this means living out the values of the kingdom of God by offering our gifts and abilities to serve others, particularly those who cannot repay us. Jesus' death and resurrection freed us not for self-serving purposes but to live lives of righteousness, which includes loving and serving others (Romans 6:16–18).

In the *ikigai* model, the overlap between what you can be paid for and what the world needs is considered a vocation. This type of work often lacks passion (*what you love*) and may not align with your natural abilities (*what you're good at*). While it serves a practical purpose, it can feel like a job done out of necessity rather than fulfillment.

I see this often with my younger clients. Many choose a career path because it offers stability—plenty of job openings and good pay. Others feel obligated to step into a family business, following a path they didn't choose for themselves. While these decisions are understandable, they can leave a person feeling unfulfilled.

As someone who once felt pressured to pursue a career that didn't align with my purpose, I know firsthand the stress and frustration it can cause. If you're a parent, leader, or mentor, guiding someone through the *ikigai* exercise is essential. Otherwise, you may unintentionally reinforce people-pleasing tendencies and contribute to their burnout. While your heart may be in the right place, truly helping others means taking the time to understand what genuinely drives them, not just what seems practical or expected.

When your work is reduced to punching a clock day in and day out for nothing more than a paycheck, it often lacks a sense of higher purpose. This emptiness can contribute to burnout, as there's no deeper connection to the work or a sense that it aligns with who you are or what truly matters to you.

To find more meaningful work, reflect on how your vocation can be enriched with passion, skill, or purpose. When all four elements of *ikigai*—what you love, what you're good at, what you can be paid for, and what for the world needs—come together, work transforms into something far more fulfilling and sustainable.

This servant-hearted approach reminds us that our freedom is not about personal gain but the opportunity to fulfill God's calling to love and care for others. When we focus on what the world needs, we align our actions with Jesus' example and embody the heart of *ikigai*, a purpose that is both meaningful and God-glorifying.

SELF-CARE PRACTICES

Nurturing your existential wellness is a vital component of self-care that connects deeply to your purpose and sense of meaning. Research shows that having a clear sense of purpose is linked to improved mental health, reduced risk of chronic disease, and greater resilience during life's challenges. By blending reflection, intentional goal-setting, and spiritual connection, you can develop a more holistic sense of *ikigai*, your reason for being, and align it with God's plan for your life.

Find your *ikigai*

Use the resources provided on this book's resources page (www.burdenedtobalancedbook.com), and start listing all the things you love, are good at, can be paid for, and are needed in the world around you. Look for overlaps to find your *ikigai*.

Reflect on your achievements

Write down your past successes, no matter how small. This can help you recognize the strengths and talents God has given you. This is one of my favorite exercises to give new clients and is supported by positive psychology. Most people do not like to brag about themselves; we want to be humble, so answering the *What am I good at?* question can be difficult for many. Spend time journaling about your successes in life and see what themes and patterns keep emerging.

Journal your goals and the reasons behind them

Setting clear, meaningful goals is scientifically proven to increase focus and achievement. Go deeper by exploring your *why*. Why is this goal important to you? Why this moment in your life? Writing about your motivations helps clarify your intentions and ensures they align with your values and faith.

Pray and meditate

These are essential practices for existential wellness, offering both spiritual and scientific benefits. Prayer invites God into your *ikigai* discovery process, providing clarity and a sense of peace. At the same time, research on mindfulness and meditation shows that these practices reduce stress, enhance focus, and foster emotional regulation. As you pray over your goals, meditate on scriptures such as Ephesians 2:10, "For we are His workmanship, created in Christ Jesus for good works, which God prepared beforehand, that we should walk in them" (ESV). This verse is a powerful reminder that your purpose is divinely designed and meant to serve a greater good.

Engage with your faith community

If it were not for my involvement in my Bible study or attending a women's retreat, this book would have never happened. Getting involved in your community can further enhance your sense of purpose. Attending religious events, such as church services or small groups, provides social connection and opportunities to deepen your understanding of God's plan. Volunteering within your community fulfills the *ikigai* element of addressing what the world needs and reinforces the biblical call to serve others. Research confirms that altruistic acts increase happiness and life satisfaction, aligning with Jesus's example of servant-hearted leadership.

By taking these steps, you create a purposeful life that integrates faith, science, and service. This holistic approach to self-care fosters a sense of fulfillment and aligns your actions with both your *ikigai* and God's greater plan for your life.

One of my favorite verses and my personal daily affirmation is Jeremiah 29:11, "For I know the plans I have for you ... plans to prosper you and not to harm you, plans to give you hope and a future." The entire verse and more are below. Spend time reading and reflecting on it.

> **Jeremiah 29:11-13**: "'For I know the *plans* I have for you,' declares the LORD, plans to **prosper** you and not to harm you, **plans** to give you **hope** and a **future**. Then you will call on me and come and pray to me, and I will listen to you. You will seek me and find me when you seek me with **all your heart**'" (emphasis mine).

Chapter Three
Mental Wellness

What do you think of when you hear about mental health? Does your mind rush to issues like depression or anxiety? Sadness or loneliness? This is what most people think of when asked about mental health. Topics such as sadness, happiness, loneliness, and anxiety will be covered under emotional wellness in the next chapter. For the purposes of this book, we will define mental health as the capacity for optimal cognitive functioning characterized by the ability to think clearly, solve problems effectively, retain memories, and focus on tasks with sustained attention. This helps us with daily tasks like trying to solve problems, puzzle piece the schedule together, or remain mindful in the moment. How many times have you jumped in the car, pulled out of your driveway, and then zoned out? You started thinking about your meetings, phone calls, or something else and the next thing you knew, you were parking at the office. When I do this, I always ask myself, *I wonder if I ran any red lights*? My body was on full autopilot driving my daily commute while my mind was thinking about other tasks entirely. Having strong cognitive health involves maintaining mental clarity, navigating challenges through logical reasoning, and managing distractions to achieve goals. Our mental health plays a vital role in our daily lives, and we must be proactive in protecting and enhancing our cognitive abilities as we age.

In my coaching practice, I use a cognitive flexibility assessment to help clients evaluate how adaptable they are to change. This assessment consists of twelve questions, measured on a sliding scale from strongly disagree to strongly agree, that explore their current beliefs. Some of the key questions are in the form of statements like, "I can find workable solutions to seemingly unsolvable problems" and "I am willing to work at creative solutions to problems." A copy of this assessment is available in this book's resource section at www.burdenedtobalancedbook.com.

This assessment is a critical tool in my coaching process because adaptability is at the heart of sustainable change. When clients come to me, they're often working to shift their habits around exercise, nutrition, sleep, and stress management. Their ability to embrace these changes directly impacts their success. Those with strong cognitive flexibility are better equipped to navigate obstacles, while those with lower flexibility may need extra support in problem-solving and developing creative solutions when setbacks arise.

Cognitive flexibility is the ability to shift between thoughts, concepts, or behaviors in response to changing situations.[v] It's a key skill for decision-making, creativity, and overall learning, especially in today's fast-paced world. As Canadian Prime Minister Justin Trudeau put it, "The pace of change has never been this fast, yet it will never be this slow again."[vi] Strengthening cognitive flexibility helps us manage uncertainty, adapt to new challenges, and ultimately, thrive in the midst of change.

Since the 2020 pandemic, I've been part of many discussions about the connection between mental resilience and cognitive flexibility. Before the pandemic, most psychologists and researchers primarily studied cognitive flexibility in relation to academic performance and creativity. However, new research is now highlighting its role in mental resilience, particularly in managing stress and reducing age-related cognitive decline. With the rise of Positive Psychology and the profound impact of the pandemic, cognitive flexibility is being recognized as a crucial factor in personal development, not just an academic concept.

We now know that individuals with higher cognitive flexibility are better equipped to handle complex or stressful situations. Their ability to shift perspectives allows them to find creative solutions and avoid rigid thinking. A simple yet relatable example is when a child unexpectedly gets sick and needs to stay home from school. A parent with strong cognitive flexibility will quickly adapt, shifting between work and caregiving responsibilities without becoming overwhelmed. That parent might rearrange their schedule, take meetings during nap time, or delegate tasks to coworkers, finding ways to meet both their child's needs and work obligations.

On the other hand, a parent with lower cognitive flexibility may struggle to adjust. That parent might feel stuck trying to adhere to the original work plan, leading to frustration, stress, and a higher likelihood of missing deadlines or neglecting the child's needs. The ability to pivot, embrace new challenges, and think creatively allows the cognitively flexible parent to navigate both responsibilities more effectively, reducing stress and maintaining balance.

Cognitive flexibility becomes increasingly important as we age, yet it naturally tends to decline over time. Fortunately, we can actively strengthen this ability through intentional cognitive training. Activities such as mindfulness practices, Sudoku puzzles, crosswords, and computer-based brain training programs help keep the mind sharp and adaptable, preserving cognitive health well into older adulthood. Taking a proactive approach to mental agility not only enhances daily problem-solving and decision-making but also serves as a protective factor against cognitive decline. Research suggests that regularly engaging in these exercises can help delay the onset of conditions like dementia and Alzheimer's disease, where a diminished ability to adapt can significantly impact quality of life.[vii] Just as we prioritize physical health through exercise and nutrition, maintaining cognitive flexibility is an essential part of lifelong well-being.

While science provides valuable insights into cognitive health, learning, and problem-solving, as Christians, we recognize that these principles are also deeply rooted in our faith. We don't rely solely on scientific evidence to understand their significance—scripture has long emphasized the importance of a sound mind and wise decision-making in our walk with Christ. The Bible reminds us that nurturing our mental well-being and seeking wisdom are not just beneficial but essential to living a life that reflects God's purpose. Our faith calls us to pursue knowledge, but more importantly, to apply it with discernment and perseverance, trusting in God's guidance. In this way, learning and problem-solving become acts of spiritual stewardship, honoring the intelligence and understanding that God has entrusted to us.

King Solomon wrote most of the book of Proverbs to teach us how to attain wisdom and apply this divine wisdom to our daily lives for our well-being. King Solomon was David's son and was known as a wise king. In 1 Kings 4:29-30 it is written, "God gave Solomon wisdom and very great insight, and a breadth of understanding as measureless as the sand on the seashore. Solomon's wisdom was greater than the wisdom of all the people of the East, and greater than all the wisdom of Egypt." This book was written so that others could embrace learning and be wise; a key verse that summarizes what we should believe about wisdom is Proverbs 1:7, "The fear of the Lord is the beginning of knowledge, but fools despise wisdom and instruction." Proverbs 1:5-6 states, "A wise man will hear and increase learning, and a man of understanding will attain wise counsel for understanding proverbs and parables, the sayings and riddles of the wise" (NASB).

The call to continuous learning is woven throughout both the Old and New Testaments. In the Old Testament, gaining wisdom was seen as essential, while in the New Testament, Jesus frequently taught through parables, challenging his followers to think deeply, ask questions, and seek greater understanding.

Those who kept their minds open and engaged were able to grasp his teachings and receive the gift of salvation. Just as cognitive flexibility helps us adapt and grow, a spiritually flexible mindset allows us to deepen our faith, respond to challenges with wisdom, and embrace the path God has set before us.

The importance of cognitive flexibility is not just a discussion for an aging population but also for our children. Children ages three to five years old undergo significant development in their cognitive flexibility, contributing to better learning outcomes and problem-solving abilities. With this significant development, we have to ask, what are we exposing our children to at such young ages? We are now seeing the effect of screen time on brain development. Studies have shown that increased screen time in young children is linked to lower white matter integrity in the brain, which can negatively affect cognitive function, language development, and literacy skills. A 2019 study found that children aged three to five who exceeded the recommended screen time had reduced white matter integrity, while more reading time was associated with better white matter organization. Additionally, research published in JAMA Pediatrics in 2019 found that higher screen usage was correlated with lower early literacy skills in preschoolers. The World Health Organization advises limiting screen time for 3- to 4-year-olds to no more than sixty minutes per day.[viiiix]

Our young children are impressionable and will mimic what they see. We must set the standards for our children. Proverbs 22:6 tells us to "Start children off on the way they should go, and even when they are old they will not turn from it." We are instructed to learn, continue our learning, and then teach our children. Instilling a sense of wonder and encouraging a love of learning, problem-solving, and exploration is easy in young children. Young children, by their very nature, are explorers and little scientists. Babies examine everything they can get their little fingers on: touching, tasting, hearing, and smelling. Babies use all their senses to explore the world around them. The hard part is keeping that wonder and love of learning alive as they grow older. This is where your habits as a mentor and guide come into play.

No matter if you are a parent, grandparent, mentor, or guide, our lives are fast paced, constantly changing, and stressful. That stress profoundly impacts our cognitive health, often disrupting our ability to learn, remember, and concentrate, which then causes more stress and compounds the issue. Much like the chicken and the egg argument about which came first: poor cognitive health or stress? In the short term, stress from daily challenges—like an argument or a looming deadline—can make us flustered and temporarily reduce the brain's ability to focus, making it difficult to process information or complete tasks efficiently. Short-term stress is expected in our day-to-day lives. However, chronic stress poses more severe risks, leading to long-term cognitive decline. Prolonged exposure to stress can cause brain regions associated with cognitive function to physically shrink, impairing skills such as attention, working memory, and cognitive flexibility.

Over time, prolonged stress may lead to brain fog, decision-making difficulties, and an inability to concentrate. Jesus never promised an easy life and following him is not always simple, especially because we are not perfect. This is where you need to give yourself grace, as Jesus knows resisting temptation gets more difficult when our cognitive health is drained. In Matthew 26:41, his disciples were fatigued and stressed from the day's activities, and Jesus warned them to "Watch and pray so that you will not fall into temptation. *The spirit is willing, but the flesh is weak*" (emphasis mine). We must take time for rest and recovery to preserve our health and remain strong. Stress encountered at crucial points in life can have lasting effects that contribute to cognitive impairment later in life, underscoring the critical need to practice stress management and self-care strategies to preserve our cognitive health.

SELF-CARE PRACTICES

Developing self-care habits to improve mental health might seem like a difficult task. How do we rest *and* exercise our brains? Unlike the other areas of wellness that we cover in this book, mental health exercises are actually some of my favorites. These practices are not only manageable but also enjoyable to put into practice. Examples of ways you can improve your mental health include:

Gratitude journaling

I cannot underscore the importance of gratitude practices. Research is very clear on how beneficial it is to establish a gratitude practice. Practicing gratitude has been shown to improve brain health by enhancing cognitive function, particularly by increasing activity in the prefrontal cortex, which is responsible for focus, decision-making, and higher-level thinking. It can also promote better sleep quality by reducing stress and fostering relaxation, essential for cognitive restoration. Additionally, gratitude boosts resilience, helping individuals navigate challenges more effectively. Regular gratitude practice positively influences key brain areas like the hypothalamus and anterior cingulate cortex, supporting both emotional and cognitive well-being.

There are many areas in scripture where we are called to practice gratitude and thanksgiving. I was taught that when a concept or story is repeated throughout the Bible, it is intended to magnify its significance, implying that we should take special notice of its meaning and how it applies to our lives. This repetition emphasizes key themes and truths that God wants us to fully grasp and reflect on, encouraging us to have a deep understanding of how to live out His message. Feel free to pick your favorite for an affirmation for daily life.

- 1 Thessalonians 5:18, "*Give thanks* in all circumstances; for this is God's will for you in Christ Jesus."*
- Colossians 3:15, "Let the peace of Christ rule in your hearts, since as members of one body you were called to peace. *And be thankful.*"*
- Psalm 100:4, "Enter his gates with *thanksgiving* and his courts with praise; *give thanks* to him and praise his name."*
- Daniel 2:23, "I *thank* and praise you, God of my ancestors: You have given me *wisdom* and power" *(emphases mine).

When practicing gratitude and journaling, understand that it is more than writing down three things you are grateful for and moving on with your day. Ask yourself, out of everything in the world, what am I most grateful for in this moment? Write it down. Then ask yourself, why, out of everything in the entire world, did I choose to write that down? Repeat this and make a list of the three to five things you are most grateful for in the moment. Spend some time, reflect on your choices, and take note that those items might change day to day.

Journal your wins

We can get in our heads about all the things we have to do, want to do, should do, or should have done already. There are many times we tell ourselves there are not enough hours in the day. This is your chance to give yourself grace. Celebrate three to five things you accomplished today. Getting yourself out of bed, finishing that project, keeping the kids alive for another day. These are things we might overlook and not give ourselves credit for accomplishing. Close each night by asking yourself, what did I accomplish today? God asks us to reflect on what is good and give thanks for what we have. In James 1:16, we are instructed to examine each achievement and blessing and thank God for what he has given us, "Every good and perfect gift is from above, coming down from the Father of the heavenly lights, who does not change like shifting shadows." Hold on to this truth and go to bed at peace, knowing that you are blessed.

Practice real meditation

My life changed when I learned how to meditate correctly. When most people think of meditation, they believe they are supposed to sit in a quiet room with their legs crossed and clear their mind of all thoughts completely. This is what I believed meditation was and as a person with diagnosed ADHD, shutting off my mind seems like an impossible task. Then, I learned how to really meditate, and it changed everything for me. When you meditate, focus on one thing. Some people focus on breathing in through their nose and out through their mouth. Others may focus on a positive affirmation or a Bible verse. One of my favorite verses to meditate on is Psalm 46:10, "Be still, and know that I am God." It helps me to remember this is a time for stillness and that God is in control; I can take my time here. As you meditate on this, other thoughts will pop into your head, but that is OK. When you catch yourself following these new thoughts, remind yourself to refocus and return to your breath, affirmation, or Bible verse. As you practice this more, you will find yourself able to catch your mind wandering quickly. This exercise has helped me to catch myself during the day when I become distracted.

This is also a wonderful practice for those in the Christian faith because it helps remind us that God is always with us. In the Bible, we are instructed to pray and meditate. Prayer involves spending time talking to God and thanking him for all he has done and casting our burdens on him, while meditation involves soaking in his presence and listening to him. There is a popular quote by Mother Teresa, "God speaks in the silence of the heart. Listening is the beginning of prayer."[x] Spend time in this practice before or after you pray and leave space for God to speak to you.

I want to acknowledge some controversy surrounding meditation among particular people of faith. I did not learn how to meditate properly for many years because I grew up in a church that had mixed opinions on the subject, so it was not discussed or taught. It is important to know that we are called to meditate, especially on the word of God. In Joshua 1:8, we are instructed to "Keep this Book of the Law always on your lips; meditate on it day and night, so that you may be careful to do everything written in it. Then you will be prosperous and successful." We should meditate as David did in Psalm 143:5, "I remember the days of long ago; I meditate on all your works and consider what your hands have done." We should meditate on God's word, consider all he has done for us, and be still so that we can hear him speak to us. Practicing meditation can alleviate our stress and reconnect us with the Father in a very powerful and intimate way.

Play more

Crossword, Sudoku, Wordle, riddles, chess, or trivia games are fun to play with the family, and all of these are great options for training your brain. Regularly engaging in puzzles, such as crosswords and jigsaw puzzles, can help slow cognitive decline and delay the onset of memory loss in older adults. Puzzles stimulate various brain regions, promoting new neural connections and improving cognitive functions like memory, attention, and processing speed, making them a valuable part of a holistic approach to maintaining brain health.

Keep learning

Read, take a course, join a Bible study or engage in intellectual debate. Research shows that participating in learning activities can greatly improve cognitive health, particularly as we get older, by promoting neuroplasticity and building cognitive reserve.[xixii] These activities help to stimulate the brain, delay cognitive decline, and reduce the risk of dementia. Reading to your children, especially from the Bible, will teach them the ways you want them to follow as they grow older while also assisting with their rapidly developing brains. Engaging in a variety of learning experiences, along with the social interaction they often provide, is crucial for maintaining cognitive function throughout life.

Let me close this chapter with a prayer from me to you. This is the same prayer Paul wrote to the church of Colossae in 60 AD:

> We continually ask God to fill you with the **knowledge** of his will through all the **wisdom** and **understanding** that the Spirit gives, so that you may <u>live a life worthy</u> of the Lord and please him in every way: bearing fruit in every good work, growing in the **knowledge** of God, being strengthened with all power according to his glorious might so that you may have great endurance and patience, and giving <u>joyful thanks</u> to the Father, who has qualified you to share in the inheritance of his holy people in the kingdom of light (Colossians 1:9-13, emphasis mine).

Chapter Four
Emotional Wellness

Mental and emotional wellness sometimes blend together, but I prefer to treat them separately. While one wellness area may affect another it is important to look at each individually. It may be difficult for some people, but it is crucial to discuss emotional wellness, what it is, why it matters, and how it impacts so many areas of our health and well-being. Simply put, emotional wellness is about understanding, managing, and expressing your emotions in a way that's healthy and productive. We need to be aware of our emotions, accept them without judgment, and use that awareness to navigate life's challenges. This does not mean being happy all the time. Good emotional wellness means you feel a wide range of emotions and you are never stuck in one single emotion.

When a loved one passes away, it is healthy to feel sadness, loneliness, grief, anger, and fear. We all need time to process the trauma of losing someone close to us. Problems with emotional health start, however, when we feel stuck. If you have a hard time moving past the grief or anger you feel, or when you no longer feel positive emotions like joy, calmness, and happiness, it can be a sign of an emotional problem.

The converse is true as well. If you feel nothing but joy—like you are on cloud nine, and you just don't come down from that feeling—it can also be a sign of emotional distress or deregulation. Our existence is messy and filled with ups and downs, and our emotions should ebb and flow with us. Good emotional wellness means accepting our feelings and not forcing specific emotions onto ourselves or others.

An example of this is toxic positivity. Toxic positivity occurs when we try to force positive emotions when we are not actually feeling positive. It is a deliberate attempt to feel joyful, causing us to ignore or dismiss our negative emotions. It is the idea to "fake it until you make it." If you find yourself plastering on a fake smile to appease those around you, you might be engaging in toxic positivity, which can have negative consequences to other areas of your health and well-being. The pressure to be happy all the time can cause guilt or shame when you legitimately feel sad, angry, or stressed; this all leads to emotional isolation or frustration.

I experienced this firsthand when I worked in the oil and gas industry. There was so much to learn about drill site safety, oversized load trucking regulations, and more—it was overwhelming. I was constantly nervous about making mistakes and struggled with confidence. I felt anxious and on edge most days, and the tension I felt caused muscle soreness and fatigue throughout my whole body. Despite those feelings, I tried my best to "fake it until I made it." Instead of talking to anyone about my fears or showing my lack of confidence, I held my head high and pushed my fears down. In a male-dominated field, the last thing I wanted was to be seen as ignorant or weak. So, I worked hard to maintain a confident and upbeat demeanor, even when I felt anything but.

Keeping up a cheerful facade increases our stress, which can make us feel burned out. Which is exactly what I did working in the oil and gas industry. Chronic stress and burnout have physical effects on our bodies. When under stress, our bodies release hormones like adrenaline and cortisol to help our hearts beat faster, muscles tighten, the digestive system slows down, and our other senses become sharper. This is a survival tactic. When faced with a predator like a lion, this is how I want my body to respond as I enter fight-or-flight mode. These are all the things I need my body to do to survive a matchup in a physically threatening situation.

Unlike our ancestors, many of us are not being chased by a lion on our way to the grocery store or work, but we all experience highly stressful situations and combat chronic stress in daily life. This comes primarily from social stress, which we will address more in the relationships chapter. Because of the increase in chronic stress illnesses, such as stomach ulcers, heart disease, hypertension, and diabetes, many articles have been published studying and discussing stress management and burnout.

I want to be clear that chronic stress and burnout are not the same thing. While they might seem similar, they're actually quite different. Chronic stress keeps you in a constant state of tension—your mind is racing, you feel overwhelmed, and everything feels like too much, but you're still pushing through. Burnout happens when that stress becomes too much for too long and completely drains you. Unlike chronic stress, which may still allow you to function, burnout makes it hard to find meaning in anything, even the things you once loved. It creates emotional detachment and an increasing sense of hopelessness. Burnout isn't just exhaustion; it's a full mental, physical, and emotional shutdown. You don't just feel overloaded; you feel empty. Stress makes you feel like you have too much on your plate; burnout makes you wonder if you even care anymore. If you want to check your current stress levels, you can find a Perceived Stress Survey on this book's resources page at www.burdenedtobalancedbook.com.

Some articles and Google searches will tell you that women experience burnout at a greater rate than men. However, a meta-analysis of gender differences in burnout by Drake University researchers Radostina K. Purvanova and John P. Muros shows that the popular belief that women experience burnout more than men is largely unsupported regarding work-related burnout.[xiii] Women may experience higher levels of emotional exhaustion, while men tend to experience more depersonalization, which is a dissociative state in which a person feels disconnected from themselves or their surroundings. It may include a sense of unreality or feeling detached from one's own thoughts, emotions, or actions as if they are observing themselves from the outside.

So, while women may become more emotionally burned out, men may become more numb and less outspoken, leaving us to believe burnout is a more prevalent issue for women than it is for men. However, burnout could be a more significant issue for men than women. If we continue to dig into the data, we find that depersonalization is linked with a higher risk of suicidal ideation.[xiv] This increased risk might explain why, according to statistics, men are 3.85 times more likely to attempt suicide compared to women.

Focusing on our emotional well-being is vital to our overall health and longevity. People with high emotional wellness can better manage their stress, form meaningful relationships, show resilience in the face of adversity, and maintain a positive outlook on life. Positive emotional wellness starts by being open and honest about our feelings. There is a misbelief that, as Christians, we are to be happy all the time. I believe the Bible verse Philippians 4:4, "Rejoice in the Lord always; again, I will say, rejoice" (ESV) is misconstrued to mean we are to be happy always.

Jesus told us that "In this world, you will have trouble" (John 16:33). He knows we will be frustrated, anxious, sad, and happy. He knows we are meant to experience many emotions but does not want us to be stuck in them. "Jesus wept," the shortest verse in the Bible, is found in John 11:35. This verse shows us it is OK to feel sad. This verse comes after Jesus learns of his good friend Lazarus's death. When Jesus saw all the people mourning over Lazarus's death, he, too, wept openly.

Having worked with many men in blue-collar industries like manufacturing, construction, and oil and gas, I know that talking about emotions can feel taboo. Many people struggle with feeling lost or emotionally drained but stay silent out of fear of being seen as weak or soft.

During a wellness-day event for a group of construction workers, I was speaking about suicide prevention and emotional well-being, encouraging the men in the room to reach out for help. I shared resources, including their employer's Employee Assistance Program (EAP), but I could feel the room disengaging. Then, one man stood up and said, "Guys, I'll be honest. I have called our EAP for myself and my sixteen-year-old son." In that moment, everything shifted. Walls came down, and men started opening up about their struggles. It was a powerful reminder that sometimes, it only takes one brave person to speak up and share their experience to create a ripple effect that impacts so many.

We are made in God's image, meaning our attributes come from our creator. There are many times in scripture where we see or are told about God's emotions. As early as Genesis 6:6, "The Lord was sorry that He had made man on the earth, and He was grieved in His heart" (ESV). Our God was sad when humankind sinned, much like a parent is sad when their child is in trouble. God can be jealous, especially *for* us, and angry toward those who sin. We see this clearly in the Old Testament, Deuteronomy 6:15, "For the Lord your God in your midst is a jealous God—lest the anger of the Lord your God be kindled against you, and he destroy you" (ESV).

Feeling specific emotions is not wrong, but when we are stuck in an emotion, it starts to destroy other areas of well-being. The top reported negative emotions in 2022 were depression and anxiety. According to the American Psychological Association, about 37 percent of adults reported having a diagnosed mental condition. This report shows a 5 percent increase from 2019, which is pre-pandemic.[xv] Of those surveyed, 24 percent cited anxiety disorder and 23 percent cited depression as their issues. Our creator knew that feelings of fear and anxiousness would be challenging to control on our own, which is why topics such as worry, fear, and anxiety appear frequently in the Bible. Depending on your translation, "Fear" is referenced over three hundred times.[xvi]

Much like stress, fear is often seen as a negative emotion, something to be avoided or eliminated. But fear, like all emotions, serves a purpose. It's not an enemy; it's a guide. In Gavin de Becker's *The Gift of Fear*, he explains how fear is a survival signal, an instinct that helps us recognize danger and protect ourselves.[xvii] From a psychological standpoint, fear heightens our awareness, sharpens our instincts, and prompts us to take action when necessary. In the Bible, fear is often a call to examine our faith, revealing where we may lack trust in God. Proverbs 9:10 tells us, "The fear of the Lord is the beginning of wisdom," reminding us that fear isn't always about danger—it can also be a reverence that leads to deeper understanding. Rather than rejecting fear, we should learn to listen to it, discerning when it's a protective warning and when it's an invitation to strengthen our faith.

SELF-CARE PRACTICES

Is there something you are feeling worried or anxious about? Starting something new like a job or moving to a new location can increase fear and anxiety. Maybe you are worried about losing a job, or you are pregnant and worried about the health and well-being of your baby. There are so many things in the world that can cause us to become worried and anxious, which is why it is essential to focus on our emotional well-being daily. Just like other areas of health, it takes continued effort to work on your emotional well-being. You cannot just do a few breathing exercises and call it a day. Here are some ways to practice emotional self-care to maintain good emotional health.

Labeling

You need to name the emotion to tame the emotion. Have you ever had someone say something to you that just got under your skin? Maybe it was passive-aggressive, and you shrugged it off at first, but later, you find yourself tossing and turning at night, unable to get the situation out of your head. This uneasiness comes from not properly naming the emotions you feel and why you feel them. Take time to walk through the situation and state out loud how it made you feel and why you feel that way.

Example of labeling: You had a stressful day at work, filled with back-to-back meetings and a tense disagreement with your manager. When you get home, you snap at your child over something small—like leaving dishes in the sink. Your child looks at you surprised, and you immediately feel guilty, unsure why you are overreacting.

Taking a moment to reflect, you realize you are not actually angry about the dishes. You are overwhelmed and frustrated from the workday, and naming that feeling of *frustration* helps you to understand why you lashed out. Once you acknowledge that you are feeling frustrated and stressed, not truly angry at your child, you feel a sense of relief. By naming the emotion, you can communicate more calmly and explain why you are on edge, which helps you better manage and "tame" the situation. Then you can explain to your child what happened, apologize, and show them how they can handle emotions when they happen.

I like how Proverbs 19:11 is written in the ESV, "Good sense makes one slow to anger, and it is his glory to overlook an offense." This proverb written by King Solomon demonstrates how it is better to ignore insults than to react to them instinctively, which can escalate the situation. A wise person defuses it by remaining calm, thinking rationally, and taming the emotion before responding. Practicing self-control can keep you out of trouble and maintain peace in your life. The concept of controlling your anger is a common theme in Solomon's proverbs.

The theme of controlling anger is so common in Solomon's Proverbs because, when left unchecked, anger leads to destructive consequences—both personally and relationally. Proverbs is a book of wisdom designed to teach people how to live righteously, make sound decisions, and cultivate strong character. Since anger is one of the most powerful and potentially harmful emotions, Solomon repeatedly warns against it and offers wisdom on how to manage it. One warning comes in Proverbs 14:29, "Whoever is slow to anger has great understanding, but he who has a hasty temper exalts folly" (ESV). Here, Solomon reminds us of the importance of pausing—taking a deep breath and thinking before we speak—especially in the heat of the moment. He also warns against surrounding ourselves with those who fuel anger and conflict. In Proverbs 22:24-25, he writes, "Do not make friends with a hot-tempered person, do not associate with one easily angered, or you may learn their ways and get yourself ensnared." His message is clear: anger is contagious, and the company we keep influences our own emotional responses. By practicing patience and being mindful of the environments we engage in, we can learn to control anger before it controls us. We will explore this further in the relational chapter, where we discuss how our relationships shape our emotional well-being.

Talk to a friend or a counselor

Pick up the phone and call a trusted friend, find time to vent to your spouse, or, if needed, schedule a session with a counselor. Talking through the situation might help you better understand the emotions you feel. Sometimes, we need a friend just to tell us our feelings are valid. Other times, we may not understand how we feel, so seeking guidance from a counselor can help determine if our feelings are healthy and how to deal with those emotions.

In Isaiah 9:6, Jesus is described as the "Wonderful Counselor." Jesus is there waiting for you to come to him and discuss what is troubling you. Paul wrote in his letter to the people of Philippi, "Do not be anxious about anything, but in every situation, by prayer and petition, with thanksgiving, present your requests to God. And the peace of God, which transcends all understanding, will guard your hearts and your minds in Christ Jesus" (Philippians 4:6-7). This is one of my favorite Bible verses.

This is not to say that feeling anxious is sinful; sometimes, this verse gets misunderstood, and you might hear messages like "worry is a sin." Being worried is not sinful in itself but getting stuck and almost obsessed with worry can be. In those times when you are feeling anxious, Paul encourages you to stop and pray. Notice the word "Thanksgiving," the practice of gratitude, showing up again in scripture. Paul clearly instructs that when you are troubled, you should stop and prepare to spend time with God. Then, with a thankful heart, remember all the times you have struggled in the past, recall how God helped you overcome those situations, and present your request to God. Remembering all that he has done for you in the past will help give you the boldness and clarity to present your troubles to Him.

Starting a business is not easy, and it's not for everyone. There's a lot of risk involved, especially when others depend on you. When I made the bold decision to leave steady employment to focus on my own business, I was filled with worry and anxiety. *Would the business succeed? Will I make enough to support my family?* Doubt, fear, and uncertainty flooded my mind. That's when I leaned even harder into scripture and deepened my prayer life. I also sought guidance from a business coach. I started working with coaches in California, where we built our businesses under the mentorship of a seasoned leader. That experience taught me an important lesson: even coaches need coaches. Reaching out for help and surrendering my worries to God is what got me to where I am today, and it's what led me to write this book. I hope it inspires you to take bold steps in your own journey.

Do not let worry and doubt control you and your thoughts; take action and talk to the Wonderful Counselor. When you feel scared, anxious, worried, angry, or lonely, pray. Take your concerns and cast them upon him. Solomon's Father, King David, writes in Psalms 55:22, "Cast your cares on the Lord, and he will sustain you; he will never let the righteous be shaken." Worries, self-doubt, and anxiety are not new concepts. God knows our hearts and wants us to turn to him when we are troubled.

Have fun

What brings you joy? Is it a mini concert in your parked car? Is it playing games with your kids? Is it going out to your favorite restaurant with friends? Do more of that. Life is busy and chaotic, and we need to make sure we are taking the time to experience happiness and joy. In his older age, King Solomon reflected on what he had learned in his life. In Ecclesiastes 3:4, he writes how there is a time for everything, "a time to weep and a time to laugh, a time to mourn and a time to dance." The question is, are you making time for happiness and joy in your life?

Even in some of my darkest times, I have always made it a point to stop for joy. I like to take a pause for positivity. When I worked in the oil and gas industry, we had a daily team meeting at 3:15 p.m. to discuss the next day's schedule. We would assign teams to service calls, ensure trucks were allocated, and coordinate vendor schedules. But before each meeting, we had a tradition: we stopped for a dance party. My team would gather a few minutes before the meeting, and I would put on some of our favorite music. We would sing, dance, and just laugh together. Taking just a few minutes to shake off stress helped us clear our minds and come to the meeting fresh, energized, and reinvigorated.

Ecclesiastes 3:12-13, "I know that there is nothing better for people than to be happy and to do good while they live. That each of them may eat and drink and find satisfaction in all their toil—this is the gift of God." According to this verse, we are to work hard and do good works but also to celebrate what we have been already blessed with. Joy is mentioned 242 times in the NIV Bible.[xviii] We are to experience joy. God instructs his people to engage in celebrations and festivals—see Deuteronomy 16:13-15 as an example of this. Psalms 149:3 states, "Let them praise his name with dancing and make music to him with timbrel and harp." In 2 Samuel 6:14, King David was so filled with joy and rejoicing he was described as "dancing before the Lord with all his might." So go crazy, put on your favorite tunes, and have a dance party in the kitchen while you reheat your coffee at 3 p.m. If it is something that uplifts your spirits and brings you joy, then go for it!

Get creative

Channel your emotions into a creative, unique expression. When emotions feel overwhelming, getting creative can provide a powerful outlet for processing and understanding those feelings. Some of the most profound works of music, literature, and art were born during times of emotional turmoil, serving as a reminder that creativity can transform pain, frustration, or sadness into something meaningful. Whether writing in a journal, painting, playing an instrument, or engaging in any other form of artistic expression, creativity allows us to externalize and explore our emotions, making them easier to manage. Instead of suppressing emotions, we can turn them into something productive and beautiful, finding healing in the process.

The Psalms are a collection of worship, poetry, and beautiful writings to God, for God, and about God. Many of the Psalms were written by David, most of them when he was facing his own turmoil, like when he was running from King Saul, hiding in the wilderness or after he had sinned against God. Some were written after victory over his enemies, praising God for his unwavering support and strength.

David wrote Psalm 13 at one of the lowest points in his life. When you first read it, you can hear his despair and see that he feels far from God. David is hiding in caves from his enemies and knows that he will fall to King Saul without God's intervention. Like many of us, he is impatiently waiting on God to help him and wondering why this is happening to him. If that is you, I encourage you to read Psalm 13 and highlight what resonates with you. Find encouragement in David's words, journal about them, pray about them, and keep pushing ahead.

I will close this chapter with a Bible verse I read weekly. This verse is about worry, reminding me not to worry about trivial things and not to worry about tomorrow but to focus on today. Jesus spoke these verses to his Disciples, so observe them well. I encourage you to circle, highlight, and underline pieces that speak to you so that you can reshape your experiences with fear, worry, anxiety, and depression for improved emotional well-being.

Matthew 6:25–34, *Do Not Worry* from the words of Jesus: Therefore, I tell you, do not **worry** about your life, what you will eat or drink, or about your body, what you will wear. Is not life more than food and the body more than clothes? Look at the birds of the air; they do not sow or reap or store away in barns, and yet your heavenly Father feeds them. Are you not much more valuable than they? *Can any one of you by* **worrying** *add a single hour to your life?**

And why do you **worry** about clothes? See how the flowers of the field grow. They do not labor or spin. Yet I tell you that not even Solomon in all his splendor was dressed like one of these. If that is how God clothes the grass of the field, which is here today and tomorrow is thrown into the fire, will he not much more clothe you—you of little faith? So do not **worry**, saying, 'What shall we eat?' or 'What shall we drink?' or 'What shall we wear?' For the pagans run after all these things, and your heavenly Father knows that you need them. But seek first his kingdom and his righteousness, and all these things will be given to you as well. Therefore, do not **worry** about tomorrow, for tomorrow will **worry** about itself. *Each day has enough trouble of its own* *(NIV, emphasis mine).

Chapter Five
Physical Wellness

When discussing health and wellness, many people immediately focus on physical wellness. They often think about exercising, increasing their intake of fruits and vegetables, or trying out a new diet they saw on TV. As a certified personal trainer, health coach, nutrition coach, and self-proclaimed gym rat, I could spend considerable time talking about this aspect of wellness. However, most people know what they should do. You probably have already heard that it is important to drink water, approximately eight glasses a day. You may have heard that you should exercise about 150 minutes of moderate intensity per week, and since you were a young child, you have been told the importance of eating fruits and vegetables.

If you are like me, you can remember quoting Thumper from the 1942 Disney movie Bambi: "Eating greens is a special treat; it makes long ears and great big feet, but it sure is awful stuff to eat."[xix] As a child, I never liked vegetables, and as an adult with Crohn's disease, vegetables have been difficult for me as I need to maintain a lower-fiber diet. There were a lot of things I was taught in health and gym class about maintaining proper physical health; however, as much as we know about it, it is something many of us take for granted.

It is not until you become sick or disabled that you realize how vital your physical wellness is. Think about any time you felt really awful. All you could think about is, "I just wish I could feel better." It is not until we become sick and tired of feeling sick and tired that we finally decide to do something about it. This is one area I encourage you to be proactive and consistent. Despite what you might think, physical wellness does not require expensive supplements, drastic changes, or hours on the treadmill. Physical well-being and self-care are about making small, consistent changes to keep your body at peak performance.

One of my favorite stories in the Bible is about Elijah in 1 Kings 19. After a long day of running for his life, Elijah collapses in the shade of a bush, exhausted and overwhelmed. He calls out to God, saying he's had enough and is ready to die. It's incredibly dramatic. Then, he falls asleep.

An angel wakes him up, and when he opens his eyes, there's bread cooking over hot coals and a jar of water waiting for him. He eats, drinks, and goes back to sleep. A little while later, the angel wakes him up again, gives him more food and water, and tells him to get moving. Strengthened by rest and nourishment, Elijah is able to travel for forty days and nights.

This story is a perfect reminder that when you feel hopeless, overwhelmed, and ready to give up, maybe what you really need is a good meal and a nap. With this story in mind, I want to focus on three key areas: sleep, nutrition, and activity. I urge you to approach these topics not from a medical perspective but from a place of self-love and self-care. Remember, God has given you just one earthly body; it is the only one you will have, and it deserves to be cherished and treated with respect.

Think back to a time when you received a very precious gift. What was that gift? How did you care for it? Did you keep it in its original box because you were afraid of damaging it? How did you feel about it if it got damaged, perhaps by a sibling or friend?

The most cherished gift I ever received is a dollhouse made by my grandfather. He spent many months crafting it by hand, and it faithfully replicated my grandparents' home. The dollhouse came with little pieces of furniture made from wood and porcelain. I spent hours playing with it in my bedroom and loved it dearly.

One day, my little brother came into my room and tried to sit on the porch roof of the dollhouse, causing it to break off, splinter the wood, and damage the front of the house. I was so upset that my parents promised to try fixing it, but it was eventually put away in storage.

I still have the dollhouse and am waiting for my daughter to be old enough to appreciate it without causing any further damage. It remains a very precious gift; one I hope to pass down to my grandchildren. It means even more to me now that my grandparents have passed away.

If I feel this sentimental and upset over a Christmas gift, shouldn't I feel the same way about the gift of my physical body? I should care for my body even more than I do for the dollhouse, especially since I want to be physically present for my grandchildren. I have noticed that when my clients begin to view their physical bodies as unique, precious gifts that can never be replicated, they approach their health in a completely unique way. The mindset shifts from *I should eat better* to *I want to eat better*. Similarly, exercise transforms from a burdensome task mandated by a doctor into a celebration of what my body is capable of. Approach the following three areas of physical wellness (sleep, nutrition, and physical activity) with a mindset of keeping your precious gift safe and functioning well.

I like to start with sleep as it regulates your entire physical body. When we do not get good quality sleep, hormones like ghrelin and leptin are imbalanced. It's funny that "ghrelin" sounds like "gremlin" because it's the hormone that makes you hungry. It is also the reason your stomach growls and sends signals to the brain when it is time to eat. When we do not get enough sleep, we produce more Ghrelin in an attempt to get more food for fuel to power our bodies through the day. Following a healthy diet is nearly impossible when your hunger gremlin is angry.

Leptin also helps to regulate food but has more to do with the timing of food. Leptin will send signals to the body to regulate food intake, so you get more to power you through the busy parts of your day and less when you are winding down for sleep. Leptin is what makes you feel full, so you do not overeat. When you are sleep deprived, your leptin levels decrease, causing you to feel hungrier, leading you to biggie-size your order or go to the refrigerator for a late-night snack.

During sleep, our brain refreshes, our muscles repair, and our immune system receives a boost, among many other benefits. Rest is essential for a healthy and functioning body. Even God rested on the seventh day! If the Lord requires rest, so do we because we are created in His image. Unfortunately, many people promote a *grind-it-out* mentality, believing that *sleep is for the weak*. This idea is as far from the truth as it can be.

Research consistently highlights the vital connection between sleep and success. Adequate sleep is not just about feeling rested; it is essential for cognitive functions like memory consolidation, focus, decision-making, and overall performance. These are the very skills we rely on to excel in our careers and personal lives. Multiple studies have shown that individuals who skimp on sleep often experience lower grades in school and reduced productivity at work. When we neglect rest, we inadvertently place barriers between ourselves and our goals, making it harder to perform at our best.

Once you have your sleep habits under control, it is easier to control your nutritional health. When we are sleep-deprived, we tend to crave more of the foods that make us gain weight and feel sluggish. We go for simple carbs like bread and sugars, looking for a boost of energy to power through the day. When we wake up feeling rested, we are able to make better food choices throughout the day. It is easier to get those fruits, vegetables, and lean proteins into the diet when we are not tired or fatigued.

In Genesis 1:29, God said, "I give you every seed-bearing plant on the face of the whole earth and every tree that has fruit with seed in it. They will be yours for food." From the very beginning of creation, God ensured we were provided with proper nourishment. After forming humankind on the sixth day and giving us our purpose, He specified what we were to eat: the fruit of the plants and trees He created. These plants and trees were uniquely designed to reproduce, sustaining not only the first generation of humans but every generation to come.

This provision highlights how deeply God cares for our well-being. By creating fruits and vegetables that naturally replenish and sustain themselves, He equipped us with an ongoing source of nourishment. Over time, humanity has learned to cultivate these seeds, expanding their abundance and ensuring that each generation has access to the nutrition needed for thriving.

When we nourish our bodies with the fruits and vegetables God created, we honor His original design and care for the precious gift of our health. Eating more of these natural, life-sustaining foods is not just about fueling our bodies; it's a reminder of the thoughtful provision that has been present since the very beginning.

Once your sleep and nutrition are cared for, it is incredible how much more energy you will have and how much better you will feel. Sleep repairs damaged muscles and gives us energy. Good-quality, nourishing food keeps inflammation low, making movement easier. You will need both adequate sleep and good nutrition to start an activity routine, whether you choose a challenging lifting schedule, to train for a marathon, or want to take first place in the pickleball tournament. Movement and staying active are essential in keeping the body functioning well.

Physical activity is one of the most impactful ways to invest in your overall well-being, no matter your age. According to the CDC, regular movement promotes better physical, mental, and emotional health. For children, physical activity sharpens thinking and cognitive skills, while for adults, it reduces anxiety and depression and even helps improve sleep quality. [xx]

As we age, staying active becomes increasingly important for maintaining mental sharpness, supporting daily functionality, and reducing the risk of chronic conditions like high blood pressure, cholesterol issues, and even certain cancers. For older adults, physical activity can lower the risk of falls and hip fractures, protect bones and joints, and prevent functional limitations that might make everyday tasks like climbing stairs or grocery shopping more difficult. Activities like walking, weightlifting, and balance exercises play a key role in maintaining independence and quality of life.

The CDC study also highlights that just 150 minutes a week of moderate physical activity can significantly lower your risk for many diseases, and doing even more amplifies those benefits. Taking more steps throughout the day matters too. For adults under sixty, aiming for 8,000 to 10,000 steps per day can reduce the risk of premature death, while adults over sixty see benefits starting at 6,000 steps per day.[xxi]

No matter where you start, every small movement adds up. Even as little as ten additional minutes of moderate activity a day could prevent an estimated 110,000 deaths annually among US adults aged forty and older. So, whether it's lifting weights, going for a walk, or simply staying active around the house, every step you take is a step toward a healthier, longer life.[xxii]

One thing that has always bothered me is seeing people with strong spiritual beliefs neglect their physical well-being. They focus heavily on the soul but overlook the care of the vessel that carries it. The idea that our earthly bodies don't matter, that only our spiritual selves are significant, is a misconception that Paul directly addresses in 1 Corinthians 6:19-20, "Don't you realize that your body is the temple of the Holy Spirit, who lives in you and was given to you by God? You do not belong to yourself, for God bought you with a high price. So, you must honor God with your body."

While this passage specifically addresses sexual immorality, the underlying message extends to all aspects of how we treat our bodies. We are called to honor our bodies as temples of the Holy Spirit. Mistreating or neglecting them is not just a disservice to us; it is a failure to respect the incredible gift God has entrusted to us.

Let's revisit the analogy of giving a precious gift to put this into perspective. Think about a time you carefully searched for the perfect present for someone you cared about or someone you wanted to impress. You invested significant time, effort, and perhaps even more money than you initially planned. None of that mattered, though, because your ultimate goal was to bring joy to that person.

Now imagine their reaction was the exact opposite of what you hoped for. Instead of appreciating your thoughtful gesture, they smashed the gift, stomped on it, and discarded it without a second thought. How would you feel?

In the same way, God has given us the gift of our physical bodies. Just as we would hope for others to cherish a gift we poured our hearts into, we are called to care for the bodies He has lovingly created for us—not just for our own benefit, but as an act of gratitude and reverence for the One who gave them to us.

But God did not stop there. Through the resurrection of Jesus Christ, we were given an even greater gift: the indwelling of the Holy Spirit. Our bodies are not only physical vessels but also spiritual dwellings, sacred places where the Spirit of God resides. Just as the Ark of the Covenant was treated with reverence, awe, and great care as it carried the presence of God, so too should we treat our bodies.

Recognizing this transforms the way we view our physical selves. Our bodies are more than tools for daily life—they are sacred vessels entrusted with the presence of the Holy Spirit. By honoring and caring for them, we not only respect God's original design but also acknowledge the profound blessing and responsibility we have been given through Christ. Let us cherish our bodies as the remarkable, holy gifts they are.

We can treat our gift properly by applying some of the following practices.

Sleep Better

It is not just about the quantity of sleep but the overall quality of sleep. As a certified sleep coach, I assist clients in implementing practices to improve sleep quality. Some of the practices you can start with are:

- Create the right environment—Ensure your bedroom is dark and cool, about sixty-five degrees Fahrenheit. Remove all electronics from the bedroom, including TVs, cellphones, iPads, etc. Lastly, make sure it is comfortable—splurge on a new mattress, pillow or down comforter.

- Develop a proper sleep ritual—Do something in the evening to give you a hit of Dopamine to relax you. Two hours before bed, you should stop working and do something you enjoy. Watch a favorite show, scroll social media, call a friend, anything that brings you happiness, not anxiety. Then, one hour before bed, get away from all the blue lights. No more TV, phone, iPad, etc. Instead, read a book, do a guided meditation, take a hot shower. Do something that helps you wind down and relax to fall into a good quality deep sleep.

- Stay consistent—Going to bed at the same time each night and waking up at the same time each morning can assist your body in finding a natural circadian rhythm, making falling asleep and waking each morning much easier. Staying up late on the weekends or sleeping in can have extremely negative effects on how you feel during the work week. Consistency is key to better sleep. There is a 72-hour rule which states how you feel today is a collection of the last 72 hours. How you slept, ate, moved your body and who you talked to all affect your mood and energy. By staying consistent you can work at peak performance.

Eat Better

I encourage you to try new things and focus on eating the rainbow: different colors of fruits and vegetables. Explore the produce section of your local grocery store and see if there are any items you have yet to eat. It is easy to find recipes online, so be bold and try something new. We even see in the Bible the transformation a proper diet can make, as in Daniel 1:12-16:

> Please test your servants for ten days: Give us nothing but vegetables to eat and water to drink. Then compare our appearance with that of the young men who eat the royal food and treat your servants in accordance with what you see." So, he agreed to this and tested them for ten days.
> At the end of the ten days, they looked healthier and better nourished than any of the young men who ate the royal food. So the guard took away their choice food and the wine they were to drink and gave them vegetables instead.

Daniel chose a vegetarian diet as an act of faith and conviction to honor God. The Babylonian king's food and wine did not align with Jewish dietary laws and were often offered to false gods. To avoid defiling himself, Daniel requested permission to eat only vegetables and drink water (Daniel 1:8). Despite initial hesitation from his handlers, Daniel proposed a ten-day test to demonstrate that he could thrive without partaking in the king's provisions (Daniel 1:12).

The test proved successful, and Daniel and his friends appeared healthier and stronger than those who ate the king's rich food (Daniel 1:15). This highlights the importance of honoring God through the choices we make about what we consume. While Daniel's story doesn't prescribe a specific diet, it reminds us that our nutritional choices are part of how we care for the physical gift God has given us.

Honoring our bodies through thoughtful nutrition is an act of respect for the temple God has entrusted to us. Whether we choose vegetables, proteins, or other foods, the focus should be on nourishing our bodies intentionally and gratefully, enabling us to thrive in the purposes God has set for us.

One practice you can adopt is to HALT before eating. HALT is an acronym representing the four main reasons people eat:

H–Hungry. When we are genuinely hungry, we should eat. It is important to nourish our bodies with healthy and wholesome food that our bodies deserve.

A–Angry/Anxious. When we feel angry or anxious, we often turn to snacks for comfort. Eating can distract us and provide extra energy to cope with the situation. However, instead of reaching for food, finding alternative ways to manage your emotions is better. Consider calling a friend, journaling about your feelings, or praying. Avoid using food as a coping mechanism for anxiety.

L–Lonely/Depressed. Feeling lonely or depressed is something we all experience from time to time. We have all seen movies or TV shows where the girl, after a breakup, goes home and cries into a tub of her favorite ice cream. Sweet, sugary foods like ice cream provide a hit of dopamine, a feel-good chemical in the brain. It's natural to seek a quick fix to feel better when we are down. However, much like when we are angry or anxious, we shouldn't rely on food as a coping mechanism for our loneliness or depression. Instead, we should explore healthier ways to cope, such as going for a walk, calling a friend, reading a book, or listening to our favorite music.

T–Tired. When we are tired, our bodies often signal us to seek out food. Typically, when we feel fatigued, we crave easily digestible simple carbohydrates, which can be found in cookies, candy, and bread. Depending on your circumstances, it may be best to take a nap or go to bed. When we are exhausted late at night, we tend to make poor food choices. Instead of giving in to these cravings and staying up late to watch a movie, consider going to bed. Getting the rest you need can help prevent your body from craving unhealthy, heavily processed foods that can lead to health issues.[xxiii]

Before you eat, HALT and ask yourself why you are eating. If you are truly hungry, then enjoy your food. However, if you find yourself eating to cope with anger, anxiety, loneliness, depression, or fatigue, consider finding a more appropriate way to manage those feelings. Avoid using food as a crutch to deal with difficult situations.

Move more

Get up and get moving. We have become an extremely sedentary society. We spend a good portion of our days sitting on our butts. We sit at our computers, in meetings, in the car commuting, at the soccer game, at the table, and then lie down and go to bed. While it might feel normal, sitting for extended periods is far from healthy. Research shows that too much sitting is linked to serious health concerns, including obesity, high blood pressure, unhealthy cholesterol levels, and an increased risk of metabolic syndrome, cardiovascular disease, and even cancer. Sitting for extended periods is so harmful that the health risks can rival those of smoking or obesity.

But there's good news—even small amounts of movement can make a significant difference. Studies suggest that sixty to seventy-five minutes of moderate-intensity activity each day can counter the adverse effects of sitting. For those who are consistently active, sitting time has little impact on overall health risks. This shows that less sitting and more movement can significantly contribute to better health.

You don't have to overhaul your life to get started. Take simple steps to incorporate more movement into your day. Stand up every thirty minutes, take a quick walk during meetings, or stand while talking on the phone or watching TV. If you work at a desk, consider a standing desk or find ways to walk while you work. Even minor changes can improve muscle tone, maintain mobility, and boost energy and mental well-being—benefits that are especially important as we age.

Movement is vital, and it does not have to be intense. The key is consistency. Every small step toward less sitting and more moving is a step toward better health and a more vibrant life.

I want to share a longer passage from Timothy for your reflection. While our spiritual well-being is more important than our physical health, we cannot fully pursue our spiritual calling if we do not care for the one body we have been gifted with. We should cherish this gift and be thankful for everything our bodies are capable of, setting an example for others to follow. When our outward appearance reflects our inner selves, showing we are healthy and happy, others will notice and might even ask for our secrets. This will be your opportunity to express your gratitude and share the message that the Lord has given you a wonderful gift.

> **1 Timothy 4:1-12**: Now the Holy Spirit tells us clearly that in the last times some will turn away from the true faith; they will follow deceptive spirits and teachings that come from demons. These people are hypocrites and liars, and their consciences are dead.
>
> They will say it is wrong to be married and **wrong to eat certain foods**. *But God created those foods to be eaten with* <u>thanks</u> *by faithful people who know the truth. Since everything God created is good, we should not reject any of it but receive it with* <u>thanks</u>. *For we know it is made acceptable by the word of God and prayer.**

If you explain these things to the brothers and sisters, Timothy, you will be a worthy servant of Christ Jesus, one who is nourished by the message of faith and the good teaching you have followed. Do not waste time arguing over godless ideas and old wives' tales. Instead, train yourself to be godly. "**Physical training is good**, but training for godliness is much better, promising benefits in this life and in the life to come." This is a trustworthy saying, and everyone should accept it. This is why we work hard and continue to struggle, for our hope is in the living God, who is the Savior of all people and particularly of all believers.*
Teach these things and insist that everyone learn them. Don't let anyone think less of you because you are young. *Be an example to all believers in what you say,* **in the way you live***, in your love, your faith, and your purity* *(NLT, emphases mine).

Chapter Six
Environmental Wellness

When most people hear "environmental wellness," they might envision movements for climate change, eco-conscious practices, or even a "back-to-nature" philosophy. But environmental wellness is much more personal, practical, and accessible than that. It is not reserved for a specific ideology or way of life—it is for anyone seeking to thrive in their surroundings. Environmental wellness is one of the seven areas I focus on in my coaching because our environment can profoundly impact our health.

Environmental wellness is the concept of living in a healthy and stimulating environment that actively supports your well-being. It's about understanding how the spaces where you live, work, and relax impact your mental, physical, and emotional health. This includes everything from your home's lighting and air quality to the noise levels at your workplace or the organization of your personal space. When we talk about environmental wellness, we're talking about how we interact with the spaces we occupy every day and how we can shape them to support a happier, healthier lifestyle.

Imagine a workplace where natural light streams through windows, the air is fresh, and the layout allows for both collaboration and privacy when needed. Compare that to a dim, cramped office with constant noise, harsh fluorescent lighting, and poor ventilation. Which environment do you think fosters better productivity, focus, and well-being? The connection between our surroundings and how we feel is undeniable.

Our society has become more accustomed to being in these harsh indoor environments and that may be the reason why we see exercises like forest bathing becoming popular. Forest bathing, also known as *shinrin-yoku*, originated in Japan in the 1980s to combat tech-related burnout and encourage people to reconnect with and protect the country's forests. This practice involves putting yourself in a forest environment to experience its sights, sounds, and sensations as a form of ecotherapy. In the 1990s, Japanese researchers began studying the physical and psychological benefits of forest bathing, affirming its positive impact on health. Though *shinrin-yoku* is a Japanese term, the concept is universal; many cultures have long understood that spending time in nature is essential for well-being.[xxiv] Because of the research done on this subject, we have seen many upgrades to places of healing like hospitals, rehab centers, and nursing homes. Patients with hospital rooms with an outdoor view of a garden or green space required less pain medication and recovered better than patients without an outdoor view.

Forest bathing has recently gained popularity in the United States through social media platforms like Instagram and TikTok. Individuals and wellness influencers have shared their experiences and highlighted the benefits they've observed by spending more time outdoors, boosting the popularity of this practice and other similar activities like hiking and grounding. This trend reflects an increasing recognition of the importance of spending time in nature to enhance personal health and well-being.

I grew up in a wooded area where my parents owned several acres they shared with deer, bears, turkeys, and coyotes. My family and I spent a lot of time in the woods, and forest rangers trained me on what to do if I ever encountered a bear while riding my dirt bike or hiking. My father was a hunter who enjoyed being outdoors, and my parents owned a hunting camp. I spent much of my time exploring the forests, floating down creeks, and building stick forts. As an adult, I was surprised to learn that "forest bathing" is an actual practice that is gaining popularity as it was a natural way of living for me. However, the more I talked to others about it, the more I realized how many people do not spend time outside in general.

I've noticed that my demeanor changes during the winter months when I spend less time outside. I somehow feel both anxious and lethargic at the same time. When the temperature drops, I make a point to counteract the effects by spending time in the sauna at the gym, getting a short UV boost from a tanning bed, or traveling south when my schedule allows. I've become very attuned to how my environment affects me, which made me curious about how others often seem unaware of the impact their surroundings have on their health and well-being.

My curiosity led me to a study in England that highlighted the health and well-being benefits of spending time outdoors. This study emphasized the time individuals spent in nature rather than just living near green spaces. By analyzing data from a large and diverse sample, the study identified a "120-minute threshold." Participants who spent at least two hours a week in natural environments reported significantly higher health and well-being levels than those with little or no exposure to nature. This positive effect was evident even among individuals living in areas with limited greenery or those dealing with long-term health conditions.[xxv] This underscores the importance of intentional visits with nature—regardless of the surroundings—in promoting both mental and physical health.

As I studied the benefits of being in nature, I started to think of all the times I read that Jesus retreated to the "wilderness" or a garden to refresh himself. In Luke 5:15-16 we read, "But the news about Him was spreading *even* farther, and large crowds were gathering to hear *Him* and to be healed of their sicknesses. But *Jesus* Himself would *often* slip away to the wilderness and pray" (NASB, emphasis mine). Another example of this is in Matthew 14, after hearing about John the Baptist's death, Jesus sought solitude by the Sea of Galilee, showing the need for the peace nature provides during times of grief or challenge.

The Garden of Gethsemane is a notable location reference throughout the four gospels. Jesus's retreat to the Garden of Gethsemane before His crucifixion provides a profound example of environmental wellness to cope with intense stress and prepare for challenging events. In His most vulnerable moments, Jesus chose a natural setting, a quiet, secluded garden at the foot of the Mount of Olives, to find solace and connect deeply with God. This setting allowed Him space for prayer, reflection, and emotional processing, underscoring the role of a peaceful environment in grounding oneself during hardship.

The choice of the garden is significant for several reasons. First, it highlights how natural surroundings can serve as sanctuaries for spiritual and emotional well-being. Surrounded by olive trees and nature's calm, Jesus found an atmosphere conducive to expressing His grief and strengthening His resolve. This example emphasizes that spending time in serene outdoor spaces can offer individuals a safe environment to process their emotions and draw inner strength.

Moreover, Jesus's example illustrates that nature can be a refuge for anyone facing challenging circumstances. Just as He sought solitude in the garden to confront His fears and prepare for what lay ahead, people today can find healing and renewal in natural settings. Gethsemane shows that even in moments of overwhelming stress, we should retreat to solitary locations where we can connect with God without the constant interruptions of technology and modern living.

Being outdoors is essential for connecting with God and nature and finding rejuvenation, but environmental wellness also involves creating intentional, supportive indoor spaces. Our indoor environment can either facilitate our goals or subtly undermine them, which is why setting up spaces for success is key. For example, many people face challenges with eating healthier and managing their weight, and the layout and contents of their kitchen can have a significant impact.

One way I help clients take control of their wellness is through kitchen cleanouts. Together, we go through their pantry and refrigerator, removing foods that don't align with their health goals and replacing them with more sensible snack and meal options. This isn't just about removing temptations; it is also about making healthier choices more accessible and creating an environment that encourages long-term success. From stocking up on nutrient-dense foods to arranging items for easy access, these small but powerful changes can help create an environment that supports mindful eating and boosts confidence. By intentionally designing our spaces, both indoors and out, we can ensure they actively contribute to our overall well-being.

SELF-CARE PRACTICES

By prioritizing our environmental health, we can revitalize ourselves physically, spiritually, mentally, and emotionally. Although environmental self-care may seem like an unusual idea, embracing several of the following practices will significantly enhance how you feel.

Spend time outside

While you go about your day, take a moment to step outside and enjoy some fresh air. Consider taking a walk, having lunch at a picnic table, or moving meetings to outdoor spaces. On nice days, I like to work on my computer outside on my back deck. By bringing just my laptop with me, I eliminate distractions like piles of paperwork waiting to be filed and other electronic devices that might vibrate or ring, keeping my focus on the task at hand.

One of my favorite Psalms written by David is Psalm 23. In verses 2-3, David writes about obedience to God, saying, "He makes me lie down in green pastures, he leads me beside quiet waters, he refreshes my soul." This imagery of peaceful natural settings conveys restoration and well-being, showing how nature contributes to emotional and spiritual renewal. Nature is often used in parables and imagery to express a need for rest and recovery. You can bring some of this serenity into your workspace by changing your environment.

Eliminate distractions

Improving work environments to boost productivity often starts with minimizing distractions, which can quickly pull focus away from essential tasks. One subtle yet common distraction is the ever-present candy dish on a coworker's desk. While it may seem harmless, this simple setup can inadvertently encourage frequent, unplanned social interactions. Colleagues may stop by for a quick treat, but the candy becomes an open invitation for small talk and interruptions, breaking the rhythm of focused work. Creating dedicated spaces for breaks or setting specific times for socializing can help curb these distractions. If you enjoy having a candy dish, consider moving it to a communal break area rather than right on your desk, where it's less likely to draw a crowd during peak work times.

Another major productivity challenge is the constant stream of digital notifications. The ping of an email, a buzz from a phone, or a pop-up from a messaging app can instantly derail focus, leading to time-consuming context-switching. Studies show that it can take several minutes to regain concentration after each distraction. Time-block your schedule and turn off all your notifications. Set specific times to check your voice messages, emails, and social media. Outside those windows of time, the notifications can be turned off.

This scenario is particularly true regarding our time spent in the Word or in prayer, and it never ceases to amaze me. I often get up early in the morning to have my alone time with God, dedicating that time to scripture reading, prayer, and meditation. However, on those busy days when I feel I need this time the most, it seems like those are the mornings when my phone goes off with last-minute changes to my schedule, or it's the morning my kids decide to wake up early as well. There will always be distractions keeping you from what is important but finding ways to overcome them and seizing other opportunities to be alone with God, reading scripture, and praying are vital to your well-being. Practicing self-control and time management can help you overcome any obstacle, even on the busiest days.

Set yourself up for success

Before I start any project, I create a checklist of things I need and make sure I have the space to work. For example, if I plan a day of baking special treats for my family, I take time to review all the ingredients I will need, purchase them from the store, clean up my kitchen, and ensure I have all the tools I need to work efficiently. If you have a goal you are working on, take time to prepare and arrange for your tasks to be performed. There are several areas in the Bible where preparation is discussed. Before certain ceremonies or battles, the people are told to prepare in specific ways. Proverbs 24:27, "Put your outdoor work in order and get your fields ready; after that, build your house." This passage teaches us that we should carry out our work in its proper order. If a farmer were to build his house in the spring, he would miss the planting season and go an entire year without food.

Planning is vital as we set our goals. We should make plans and then set up our environment for our desired success. For instance, if your goal is to get a better quality of sleep each night, you can set your environment up for success by practicing the following:

- Turn electronic devices to "Do Not Disturb" mode while you prepare and plan to sleep.

- Avoid screen time one hour before bed; blue light affects our circadian rhythm.

- Make sure the room is dark. Purchase black-out curtains if needed.

- Set the temperature to a colder setting—around sixty-five degrees is the ideal temperature

- Remove all electronic devices from the bedroom: no computers, TVs, iPads, etc. Charge your devices outside the bedroom, as the frequencies can interfere with sleep patterns.

You can set up your environment in many ways to be more successful personally or professionally. This might mean a kitchen cleanout, removing the laundry from the treadmill, filing the papers, and cleaning your workspace so you can focus. Whatever it is for you, set yourself up to be successful, plan carefully, and design the space you need to succeed.

Take up gardening

It is not enough to simply enjoy nature; we are also entrusted with the responsibility to protect and nurture it. Genesis 2:15 says, "The Lord God took the man and put him in the Garden of Eden to work it and take care of it." This verse highlights that caring for the environment is a core part of living a fulfilling and purposeful life. Engaging with nature through activities like gardening not only connects us to the earth but also reduces stress and enhances mental well-being. By tending to nature, we support its growth and vitality, recognizing that our own wellness is intricately connected to the health of the environment. We are called to be stewards, benefiting from nature's gifts and actively participating in its preservation and flourishing.

If you're like me and feel you have a "black thumb" rather than a green one, simple indoor plants can still bring meaningful benefits to your home. Adding plants like Philodendrons, Spider plants, and Snake plants can have significant impacts on your health and well-being with minimal effort. These low-maintenance plants thrive indoors with the right balance of sunlight and water, and beyond being decorative, they actively improve air quality. A NASA study found that indoor plants can remove volatile organic compounds (VOCs), such as formaldehyde and carbon monoxide, which are common in household air. For instance, Spider plants were shown to remove up to 95 percent of toxic formaldehyde from the air in a sealed environment over just twenty-four hours. This natural filtering effect helps reduce pollutants, creates a fresher, healthier indoor space, and boosts mood and energy levels.[xxvi][xxvii]

As you think about how to practice environmental wellness, reflect on the one who created the environment in which we live. God created the earth, the heavens, and us. He purposely created everything and placed man in a garden to tend to it and flourish. We should regard everything that God has created as precious. Even God looked upon all He had made and saw that it was good, which means it is beneficial for us. Take a moment to meditate on the scriptures below and reflect on how you can embrace environmental wellness as part of your self-care and well-being.

> **Genesis 1:1- 2:** "In the beginning, **God created the heavens and the earth**. The earth was without form and void, and darkness was over the face of the deep. And the Spirit of God was hovering over the face of the waters. And God said, 'Let there be light,' and there was light. And God saw that *the light was good*. And God separated the light from the darkness. God called the light Day, and the darkness he called Night. And there was evening and there was morning, the first day" (emphasis mine).

Genesis 1:29-31: "And God said, 'Behold, I have given you every plant yielding seed that is on the face of all the earth, and every tree with seed in its fruit. You shall have them for food. And to every beast of the earth and to every bird of the heavens and to everything that creeps on the earth, everything that has the breath of life, I have given every green plant for food.' And it was so. And **God saw everything that he had made, and behold, *it was very good***. And there was evening and there was morning, the sixth day" (emphasis mine).

Chapter Seven
Relational Wellness

Growing up, I often heard the advice to "choose your friends wisely." At the time, I didn't fully grasp how much the people around me could influence my life. I gave little thought to the types of relationships I was building, taking them for granted. Now, as I write this chapter on relational wellness, I see those words through an entirely different lens.

Relational wellness isn't just a luxury or an afterthought—it's foundational to our well-being. Research shows that supportive relationships are powerful tools for improving mental health, enhancing resilience, and even adding years to our lives. In today's world, where connections can feel shallow and fleeting, intentionally nurturing meaningful relationships has never been more critical.

Relationships are being more thoroughly studied in the wake of the 2020 pandemic. During that time, people were forced to isolate themselves to keep the COVID-19 virus from spreading. This was exceptionally difficult for those who lived alone or were single parents with no way to get additional support. A study conducted by Harvard in 2021 found that 36 percent of Americans reported experiencing "serious loneliness" in the aftermath of the pandemic. The issue was particularly pronounced among young adults (61 percent) and mothers of young children (51 percent). While social distancing measures were necessary to control the spread of COVID-19, they significantly heightened feelings of isolation for many individuals.[xxviii] The study also explored the different types and causes of loneliness, as well as its potentially serious consequences, which can include early mortality, depression, anxiety, heart disease, and substance abuse.

Our brains are hardwired for relationships. If we take a quick look at the "triune brain" model, developed by Paul MacLean, we can better understand how and why our brains developed as they did. This model is an evolutionary theory of brain development that emphasizes three key brain regions: the basal ganglia for survival, the limbic system for connections, and the neocortex for higher problem-solving.[xxix]

First is what is known as the reptilian brain or basal ganglia. The basal ganglia region is responsible for basic survival functions like breathing, heart rate, and fight-or-flight response. It is also the part of the brain that looks for patterns like *fire means hot and it burns*, *sun goes down, moon comes up*, and *gray clouds mean rain*. It would make sense that this is the first part of our brain to develop; it also aligns with Maslow's hierarchy of needs. Maslow suggested that first, we need physiological needs such as air, water, shelter, and food. The next stage in his theory includes safety needs like personal security and resources.[xxx] The basal ganglia is about survival, and this is the portion of the brain that is looking for physiological and safety needs.

The next region of our brain to develop was the Paleomammalian brain or the limbic system. This region is responsible for emotions, memory, and social bonding. Once again, this aligns with Maslow's theory, as the next stage is love and belonging. Think about our ancestors and their evolution. First, they would be focused on survival. They would wander the savannah with a stick looking for resources when suddenly a lion jumps out at them. Their brains switch to fight or flight mode and either fight the lion off, flee from it, or die. As time progressed, they realized that when searching for resources as part of a tribe and a lion jumped out at them, their chances of survival increased exponentially. Ten people can fend off a lion much easier than one. Or should you choose to flee, you have to be faster than one other person to survive. It is natural to believe that a system would develop in our brains that would make us crave connections with others for our survival.

When I studied this model of brain development and then thought about how it related to what I was taught about creation, I noticed similar parallels. God made the earth, sky, water, and animals; on the sixth day He created man. God put man in the Garden of Eden, where he had shelter, food, and safety. This not only fulfills the first two levels of Maslow's hierarchy of needs but also explains why a man would only need his basal ganglia. Adam would look for the patterns God had made, such as the difference between day and night. What is interesting is that Genesis 2:18 says, "The Lord God said, 'It is *not good* for the man to be alone. I will make a helper suitable for him'" (author emphasis). As we read in the environmental chapter, after each day of creation, God looked upon what he created and stated it was "good" or "very good." This is the first time God looked upon what he has created and described it as "not good."

Realizing that Adam needed companionship and a helper, God created woman. In Genesis 2:22, Eve was formed from Adam's rib, a symbol of equality and partnership, designed to stand by his side. With Eve's creation, we see the fulfillment of the next stage in Maslow's hierarchy of needs: the love and belonging stage. Adam's life was no longer solitary; it now included the deep emotional connection and bonding that only companionship could bring. This transition highlights an essential human truth: relationships and community are foundational to well-being and fulfillment.

From a neurodevelopmental perspective, this aligns with the activation of Adam's limbic brain region, which governs emotions, connection, and social bonding. Just as the triune brain model suggests the limbic system evolved to enable attachment and emotional depth, Adam's newfound connection with Eve reflects this developmental progression. Together, they represent a unified whole, capable of forming bonds that go beyond survival instincts to encompass emotional intimacy and partnership.

The parallels between biblical creation, Maslow's hierarchy, and the triune brain model suggest a designed progression in human development. God provided Adam with his basic needs, shelter, safety, and sustenance, meeting his physiological and security requirements. When those needs were fulfilled, the next phase was relational, fostering the emotional depth necessary for love and belonging. This layered design mirrors both psychological theory and neurological development, demonstrating that humanity is intricately wired for growth, connection, and purpose.

The desire to belong to a tribe or community is deeply ingrained in our limbic system, as it plays a crucial role in our survival. This is why being ostracized can lead to significant stress and anxiety. If someone was part of a tribe and then cast out, their chances of surviving alone would be extremely low. Even though we no longer dwell in caves and fight lions on our way to work, that part of the brain still craves emotional connections, and not having those connections increases stress, anxiety, depression, and other health issues.

Thanks to our uniquely designed brains, our desire to be included socially is extremely powerful and can affect us not just mentally but also physically. One interesting study was performed by Eisenberger and Lieberman in 2003. In this study, they took participants into a lab, hooked them into functional magnetic resonance imaging (fMRI) brain scanners and then instructed them to play a virtual ball toss game. It was simple: while in the brain scanner, Participant A tossed the ball to Person B, who tossed it to Person C, and then they tossed it back to Participant A. Like all good psychological studies, they lied to the participants, and they were not playing with each other but a computer simulation (persons B and C). After some time had passed, Participant A would be cut out of the game. Persons B and C would toss the ball back and forth, leaving Participant A as a bench warmer on the sideline. They found that when the participant experienced social exclusion (like being left out of a virtual ball-tossing game), the same brain regions associated with physical pain activated.[xxxi]

We've all been there, receiving bad news, feeling betrayed, or being rendered an outcast by someone we trusted. When we try to describe it, we often say it felt like we were "punched in the gut." It turns out there's truth to that expression. The same neural pathways that process physical pain in the body also process social and emotional pain. This connection could help explain why so many people overuse pain medications. These medications don't just numb physical pain, like a sprained ankle; they can also dull the sting of social or emotional pain, providing temporary relief from the invisible wounds we carry.

Having a community is essential for our health and overall survival, just as it was for our ancestors thousands of years ago. It's not only important to have a community, but having the right one is crucial. The people you choose to spend time with can influence you in ways you may not even realize. Your community and friendships significantly shape your life by providing social support, influencing your values and behaviors, enhancing your sense of belonging, and impacting your overall mental and emotional well-being. Essentially, the people around you can greatly affect your outlook on life and how you navigate challenges. Proverbs 13:20 puts it simply, "Whoever walks with the wise becomes wise, but the companion of fools will suffer harm" (ESV).

The friends you surround yourself with can significantly influence your path to success. Studies have shown that spending time with successful friends can inspire you to set higher goals, work harder, and achieve more. This phenomenon, often called "social contagion," highlights how positive behaviors and attitudes can spread through social circles, fostering personal growth and achievement.[xxxii] For instance, in academic settings, students who are surrounded by high-achieving peers often see an improvement in their own academic performance. The same principle applies in other areas of life, where being in the company of driven and accomplished individuals can create a ripple effect, boosting your own aspirations and accomplishments.

I've noticed shifts in my social groups as my career has evolved. When I worked in oil and gas, I spent a lot of time in bars, hanging out with the blue-collar guys. It was fun; they were a supportive group, and I enjoyed my time with them. But as I moved into the wellness industry, my time with them became more limited, and I naturally developed a new social circle: people I exercised with, built coaching skills alongside, and swapped healthy recipes with. Even now, as I write this book, I find myself in yet another phase, spending more time with authors, speakers, and advocates.

Aligning your social groups with your goals is essential for growth. While I still keep in touch with some old friends in the oil and gas industry, I know that staying within one social circle would have limited my growth in other areas. It's like the old saying: *Make new friends but keep the old.* At the same time, I've had to be mindful of who I surround myself with. Over the years, I've had to let go of people who were toxic to my well-being and held me back. Understanding that some relationships are only meant for a season is a tough but necessary lesson if you want to keep evolving.

Having successful friends not only inspires you but also offers valuable perspectives and strategies. They bring unique insights and approaches to challenges, exposing you to new ways of thinking and problem-solving. Beyond this, their ambition can create a sense of accountability, motivating you to stay focused and push yourself further. Importantly, these friends also serve as a supportive network, celebrating your achievements, encouraging you during tough times, and bolstering your confidence and resilience.

However, the quality of these friendships matters more than their quantity. Genuine, supportive relationships with successful individuals are far more impactful than superficial connections based solely on accomplishments. It's also essential to avoid falling into comparison traps, which can lead to self-doubt. Instead, focus on learning from your friends' experiences and using their success as inspiration for your own growth. Choosing the right friends isn't just about surrounding yourself with success; it's about building a circle of trust, encouragement, and shared ambition that lifts everyone higher.

The Bible provides profound wisdom on the importance of choosing the right friends and community for positive growth. Proverbs 27:17 declares, "As iron sharpens iron, so one person sharpens another," illustrating how meaningful relationships help refine and shape us. Just as steel becomes sharper through the friction of another piece of metal, people grow and develop when they interact in ways that challenge, support, and encourage one another. This sharpening process often involves constructive conflict—Proverbs 27:6 reminds us that honest feedback, though it may be uncomfortable, is an essential part of growth, "Wounds from a friend can be trusted, but an enemy multiplies kisses." Fellow believers who avoid challenging or questioning each other risk remaining spiritually and emotionally stagnant.

The Bible also provides examples of relationships that foster growth and godliness. Jesus sent His disciples out in pairs, ensuring that each could sharpen the other's testimony. Similarly, Paul's mentoring relationship with Timothy not only strengthened Timothy's faith but also encouraged him to pass on what he had learned to others, as seen in 2 Timothy 2:2, "what you have heard from me in the presence of many witnesses entrust to faithful men, who will be able to teach others also" (ESV). The friendship between David and Jonathan further illustrates how strong relationships can provide encouragement, spiritual strength, and emotional support. Together, they shared a bond that uplifted their faith and fortified their spirits through prayer, trust, and shared purpose.

This wisdom underscores the need to choose who we surround ourselves with carefully. Proverbs warns us that ungodly companions can lead us into sin and destruction. In Proverbs 22:24–25, we are taught, "Do not make friends with a hot-tempered person, do not associate with one easily angered, or you may learn their ways and get yourself ensnared." Building relationships with godly friends can lead us toward personal growth and a stronger faith. Solomon reminds us in Proverbs 17:17, "A friend loves at all times, and a brother is born for a time of adversity." This verse highlights the profound value of true friendship and brotherhood. A genuine friend shows unwavering love, and a brother stands beside us in our hardest moments. Together, they reflect the essence of steadfast love, not only in favorable circumstances but also when life feels uncertain or challenging. When we surround ourselves with people who challenge us in love, provide wise counsel, and walk with us in faith, we create a community that strengthens our resilience, encourages our growth, and draws us closer to God.

SELF-CARE PRACTICES

Relationships, like other areas of wellness, require effort and consistent practice. I challenge you to ignore your spouse, child, or close friend for a day and see how they react. Neglecting your most important relationships can cause significant harm and could even result in losing a good friend. It's easy to get caught up in the daily grind and forget to check in with those we care about. Therefore, it's essential to develop healthy habits that strengthen our relationships. Here are some practices you should incorporate into your daily routine to maintain and nurture your relationships.

Pray daily

Your relationship with your Lord and Savior is the most important one you'll ever develop; yet, for many of us, it's the one we neglect most. Developing this relationship starts with making prayer a daily habit. One of the biggest misconceptions about prayer is that it needs to follow a strict formula filled with the "right" religious words. Many people are unsure how to pray or what to say during prayer. There is no magic formula to prayer or script you have to follow. Scripture shows us a much more personal and flexible approach to prayer, one that looks like an honest conversation between loved ones. In Exodus 3:11-14, Moses argued with God about his fears of returning to Egypt and Elijah poured out his loneliness and frustration to God in 1 Kings 19:10.

Some of my favorite prayers to read are David's because he prayed about a wide array of issues. David's prayers are powerful examples of raw, unscripted dialogue with God. He asked rhetorical questions like in Psalm 2:1, "Why do the nations conspire and the people plot in vain?" He pleaded for guidance in Psalm 5:8, "Lead me, O LORD, in your righteousness because of my enemies; make your way straight before me" (ESV). He pleaded for forgiveness after committing a great sin in Psalm 51:1, "Have mercy on me, O God, according to your unfailing love; according to your great compassion, blot out my transgressions." He also rejoiced in God's goodness, in Psalm 23:6 declaring, "Surely your goodness and love will follow me all the days of my life, and I will dwell in the house of the Lord forever."

What's striking is how David's prayers shift. In one moment, he's frustrated with the world; in another, he's crying out for personal help; and soon after, he's celebrating God's faithful love. Perhaps the most profound example of prayer's simplicity comes in Psalm 27:8, "My heart has heard you say, 'Come and talk with me.' And my heart responds, 'Lord, I am coming.'"

Prayer doesn't need to be perfect. It just needs to be honest. In Jeremiah 29:12-13, we see how God responds to our prayers. "Then you will call on me and come and pray to me, and I will listen to you. You will seek me and find me when you seek me with all your heart." As long as you are being honest and are seeking God with all your heart, he will hear your prayers, and you will find him. Take a moment each day to talk with God, whether you're celebrating, questioning, pleading, or simply showing up. The most important thing is to come.

Call a friend or family member

Just as your relationship with your Heavenly Father thrives when you devote time and attention to it, your earthly relationships need the same care to grow and flourish. The bonds we share with family and friends are not self-sustaining; they require consistent effort and intentionality. Simple, small gestures can profoundly impact both your heart and theirs.

Take a moment to call a friend or family member, even if it's just for two minutes. A brief call to say, *I just wanted you to know I'm thinking about you, and I appreciate you,* can mean the world. Those two minutes might seem insignificant, but they carry the power to ease your mind and brighten someone else's day. Relationships are built in these small, thoughtful moments, when connection triumphs over busyness.

It doesn't have to be a grand gesture. Often, it's the simplest acts of love and kindness that strengthen our relationships the most. These small efforts remind the people in your life that they matter to you and that they are seen and valued. And in return, they remind you of the joy that comes from nurturing those connections. Just as a quick prayer can center your relationship with God, a quick call can do the same for your earthly relationships. Over time, these small investments create a foundation of trust, love, and gratitude that enriches every aspect of your life.

Plan a date night

A surprising number of marriages end in divorce simply because one or both partners feel unappreciated. It's easy for time and energy to be consumed by children, careers, and other ambitions, leaving little room for each other. However, neglecting communication and quality time together can quietly erode a marriage. That's why it's so important to intentionally set aside time to reconnect with your spouse.

A date night doesn't have to be a fancy evening out, especially if finding a babysitter feels impossible. My husband and I often plan lunch dates instead. While the kids are at school and we're working from home, we'll carve out time to meet in the kitchen for a quick bite or head to our favorite Mexican restaurant. Lunch dates have their perks: they're usually more affordable, there's less stress about the kids because we know they're in school, and we're still home in time to greet them when the bus arrives. Plus, we have more energy to talk and genuinely connect during the day than we would after a long, exhausting evening.

If a lunch date doesn't work for you, call that babysitter and plan an evening out. Your kids will be fine. In fact, seeing their parents prioritize their relationship is a healthy example for them. Remember, this isn't just about spending time together; it's about showing your spouse they're still a priority. Chances are, they need that time with you just as much as you need it with them.

Write a letter

To build quality relationships, consider taking the time to write a letter to a friend or family member. Yes, it might seem old-fashioned in today's fast-paced digital world, but there's something deeply therapeutic about putting pen to paper. A handwritten note carries a sense of intention and care that a quick text or email can't replicate. It allows you to slow down, reflect, and express your thoughts in a meaningful way.

Whether it's a letter of gratitude, encouragement, or simply a heartfelt "thinking of you," this small gesture can make a big impact. For the recipient, opening a handwritten letter is a special moment that reminds them they are valued and loved. And for you, the act of writing can be a powerful reminder of the importance of nurturing your relationships. Sometimes, the most timeless practices are the ones that make the deepest connections. So, grab a pen and some paper, and take a moment to strengthen a meaningful bond.

We are created for relationships and companionship; they're woven into our very design. That's why it's so important to find your tribe or community—the people who will walk alongside you in life. But remember, just like any other area of wellness, relationships take effort and care to maintain. In today's world, messages like *I'm a strong, independent woman who doesn't need anyone* or *I'm better off on my own* are often celebrated. But don't be fooled, these are lies whispered by the one who seeks to isolate and destroy you. God created us for connection; even science confirms that our brains are hardwired for relationships and social bonds. Don't go it alone. Take a moment to reflect on the following Bible verses and consider who in your life you need to reconnect with today. Relationships are worth the work—they're part of God's plan for your joy, growth, and purpose.

Ecclesiastes 4:8-12: There was a man all **alone**; he had neither son nor brother. There was no end to his toil, yet his eyes were not content with his wealth. "For whom am I toiling," he asked, "and why am I depriving myself of enjoyment?" This too is meaningless—a miserable business!* *Two are better than one,* because they have a good return for their labor: If either of them falls down, one can help the other up. But pity anyone who falls and has **no one** to help them up.*

Also, if two lie down together, they will keep warm. But how can one keep warm **alone**? Though one may be overpowered, two can defend themselves. A cord of three strands is not quickly broken. *(emphases mine).

Chapter Eight
Financial Wellness

There are many different ideas about what it means to be financial well or financially abundant. For the purposes of this book, I view financial wellness as the ability to manage your money with confidence and feel secure about your financial future. It means meeting your current and future financial needs while making choices that allow you to enjoy life along the way. Financial wellness goes beyond just having a budget or knowing about investments; it's about managing your economic life effectively, reducing financial stress, and aligning your financial decisions with your values and goals. To understand how financial wellness is perceived in this book you can take our life balance assessment found at www.burdenedtobalancedbook.com.

Financial wellness might seem like a strange addition to the idea of deep health. However, it came up so frequently when working with clients that it only made sense for me to include it in my program. Finances impact multiple aspects of our lives, yet so many people lack financial literacy or preparation. Being unwell in this area creates a cycle of stress, affecting both their mental and physical health. When helping clients recover from burnout, I often administer the Perceived Stress Scale. For those who score in the moderate to high-stress range, the first question I ask is, "What are you most stressed about right now?" The answer is almost always the same: finances.

I wasn't the only one noticing this trend with our assessment. The 2023 PwC Employee Financial Wellness Survey revealed that 57 percent of respondents identified finances as their primary source of stress. Among full-time employees, 60 percent reported feeling stressed about their financial situation. Even those earning $100,000 or more annually were not exempt, with 47 percent expressing similar concerns.[xxxiii]

Whether clients were grappling with student loan debt, saving for their first home, preparing for a new baby, planning for a child's college education, or looking ahead to retirement, financial concerns were consistently at the top of their minds. These worries often lead to significant stress, sleepless nights, and poor nutritional habits. Food frequently became a coping mechanism for stress, compounding other health challenges. It is clear the impact of financial stress goes beyond just money; it affects mental health, sleep, and self-esteem.

Numerous studies show a strong link between financial stress and poor health. People dealing with significant financial worries are more likely to struggle with mental health issues like depression and anxiety. Financial stress also takes a toll on physical health, increasing the risk of chronic diseases and leading to poorer overall health. Those hit hardest tend to be individuals with low incomes, high levels of debt, or facing unemployment.[xxxiv]

Anyone reading this book could have dealt with financial worry at some point in their lives. We've all been there: a car breaks down unexpectedly, a home repair pops up out of nowhere, or a job loss takes us by surprise. Politicians often evoke the image of a family sitting around the kitchen table, stressing over bills, to push their economic policies. It's a scene that resonates because it's so familiar to all of us. And yet, none of these financial woes are a new concept. In the NIV version of the Bible, wealth is mentioned 126 times, money 113 times, gold 441 times, and shekels 84 times.[xxxv] The Bible has a lot to say about money and wealth.

Even though financial stress is something we all experience and understand its effects, it's the one topic most people find toughest to talk about. I'm often amazed at how open clients can be with me—they'll share their age, weight, medications, health issues, struggles with substance abuse, and even family challenges. But when the conversation turns to finances, how much they make, how much is in their bank account, or the amount of debt they have, it suddenly feels like I've crossed a line. Surprisingly, people are often more willing to discuss deeply personal matters than their financial situation. There seems to be less stigma around discussing mental health now than there is around financial topics.

Money can evoke strong emotions, particularly in the Christian community, where beliefs about finances vary widely. On one end of the spectrum, some believe God wants you to be rich, while others believe that you should live in poverty and devote everything to the Lord. These extremes and the beliefs that fall in between often lead to tension, intense feelings, and negative perceptions about money and finances.

I have heard clients use a variety of words when describing their feelings about money, including shame, guilt, embarrassment, greed, unworthiness, fear, and pride. These emotions often stem from a deep sense of inadequacy or failure, whether it feels like they haven't saved enough, made poor financial decisions, or are unable to meet societal or family expectations.

For many in the Christian community, these emotions are compounded by spiritual beliefs and teachings about money. Some of the teachings come in half-truths. Shame can arise from the assumption that financial struggles indicate a lack of faith or stewardship, as in Proverbs 22:7, warning about the dangers of debt, "The borrower is slave to the lender" (ESV). Guilt may come from feeling as though they have mismanaged God's blessings or prioritized material wealth over spiritual growth, as Matthew 6:24 reminds us, "You cannot serve both God and money."

Embarrassment might stem from financial difficulties being perceived as a failure to trust in God's provision, while greed and pride often conflict with teachings about humility and generosity, such as in 1 Timothy 6:10, "For the love of money is a root of all kinds of evil." Fear about financial uncertainty can reflect a struggle to fully embrace verses like Philippians 4:19, "And my God will meet all your needs according to the riches of his glory in Christ Jesus." Unworthiness may manifest when individuals feel they don't deserve financial stability, misinterpreting the concept of living sacrificially as living in lack.

These deeply held spiritual and emotional connections to money not only create barriers to discussing finances but also contribute to a cycle of stress and avoidance. Addressing these feelings with grace and biblical wisdom can help individuals find a healthier and more faithful relationship with their finances.

Common questions to consider: How should we view money? What should we believe about wealth? How can we practice financial wellness?

I love P.T. Barnum's quote, "Money is, in some respects, like fire. It is a very excellent servant but a terrible master."[xxxvi] This reminds me of Matthew 6:24, "No one can serve two masters. Either you will hate the one and love the other, or you will be devoted to the one and despise the other. You cannot serve both God and money." Most people focus only on the last part of the verse, but the whole passage drives home the point. As Barnum noted, money is a terrible master and treating it as one leads to frustration and even resentment.

In this world, we need money; how will I live if I don't have money? This knee-jerk reaction often arises when people read this verse. It's a natural response because wanting financial security, possessions, and enjoyable experiences is human nature. Jesus doesn't say it's wrong to desire both. What He makes clear is that we cannot give ultimate priority to both at the same time. Life often forces us to choose which is more important. Christ's calling requires us to decide whether to serve God or serve money.

Scripture uses the metaphor of servanthood: a servant cannot serve two masters equally. Loyalty will always lean toward one over the other. Jesus teaches that we are either servants of God or servants of wealth. Those devoted to money depend on it for security and fulfillment, while those devoted to God trust Him to meet all their needs. The demands of these two masters will always conflict.

Those who prioritize wealth may acknowledge God, but often only in the margins or for superficial reasons. Ultimately, there can only be one "most important" thing in our lives. This doesn't mean that serving God wholeheartedly requires avoiding money or possessions. Jesus isn't saying Christians must be poor or reject all luxury. Instead, He's teaching that a righteous person doesn't center their life on acquiring wealth. For them, money is simply a tool to be used for God's purposes.

Tools can be used for positive or for harmful purposes. A hammer can bring boards together to build incredible structures, or it can be used to break things apart and destroy what was once good. Money is no different; it's a tool. What matters is what you do with it, how you use it, and where you prioritize it in your life. For money to reach its full potential, it must be in circulation. Hoarding it serves no real purpose. What good is it doing if your money is sitting in your wallet or bank account? But when you use it—for example, by giving it to charities that provide clothing, food, and supplies to those in need—you turn it into a force for good. Like any tool, money gains its value from how it is used.

One story that illustrates this is found in Luke 12:16-24. Jesus shares a parable about a man who values his earthly wealth more than his relationship with God. This man is already wealthy, and when his field produces an abundant crop, he faces a decision. His barns are already full, but instead of using his surplus to help the poor or further God's kingdom, he chooses to stockpile his abundance and retire in comfort.

Jesus highlights several flaws in this man's plan. First, the farmer is fixated on his earthly possessions rather than the eternal kingdom God offers to those who worship Him. He fails to see that his blessings are meant to be shared and used to help others, as is taught in Hebrews 13:16, "And do not forget to do good and to share with others, for with such sacrifices God is pleased." The man also misunderstands the purpose of a faithful life, which is not about hoarding wealth or achieving early retirement but about serving God, managing His resources responsibly, and leading others with integrity. This is also taught by Jesus's disciple in 1 John 3:17, "If anyone has material possessions and sees a brother or sister in need but has no pity on them, how can the love of God be in that person?"

The man's sin is not that he is wealthy or that he has stored his grain. Instead, his attitude is one of greed. Jesus calls it "covetousness." This greed is akin to idolatry, as Paul describes in Colossians 3:5: the man places his trust in his riches instead of in God. Meanwhile, unknown to him, his life is about to end. His accumulated wealth will mean nothing. He has neglected to prioritize his eternal relationship with God, and now he must face the consequences. Jesus uses this parable to remind His followers that this is not the way they are called to live. Instead, they are to seek God's kingdom above all else.

For a long time, I had a very antagonistic relationship with money. I grew up misquoting the Bible, stating that "money is the root of all evil," and thinking about the Bible story in Matthew 19:23-26, where a man approached Jesus asking how he can get into heaven. Jesus told him to sell everything he owned and give it to the poor. The man walked away sad because he did not want to give up his possessions. Jesus then tells his disciples, "It is hard for someone who is rich to enter the kingdom of heaven. Again, I tell you, it is easier for a camel to go through the eye of a needle than for someone who is rich to enter the kingdom of God." Because I misunderstood what Jesus was teaching and my misquotes, I believed that having money and wealth was wrong.

When I started my business, I had a very difficult time asking for money. Even my clients told me I did not ask for enough, and many of them (in kindness) offered to pay me more than I quoted. I felt asking for more was being greedy. It wasn't until I started working with a Christian business coach and a sales coach that I started to learn more about these verses and their true lessons. I learned it is not a sin to be wealthy.

The Bible verses that put things into perspective more for me were 1 Timothy 6:7-10:

> For we brought nothing into the world, and we can take nothing out of it. But if we have food and clothing, we will be content with that. Those who want to get rich fall into temptation and a trap and into many foolish and harmful desires that plunge people into ruin and destruction. For the *love* of money is a root of all kinds of evil. Some people, eager for money, have wandered from the faith and pierced themselves with many griefs (emphasis mine).

Being wealthy is not the problem; not knowing when it is enough is the problem. Loving money and trusting in money *more* than God is the issue that leads to sin. This insight has been shared in the Bible and by others we may also view as successful individuals. John C. Bogle, the founder of The Vanguard Group, shared a memorable story during his commencement address for MBA graduates at Georgetown University's McDonough School of Business in May 2007. He recounted a tale involving authors Kurt Vonnegut and Joseph Heller in his speech. At a party hosted by a billionaire on Shelter Island, Vonnegut pointed out to Heller that their host, a hedge fund manager, had earned more money in a single day than Heller had made from his renowned novel *Catch-22* over its entire history. Heller's response was profound, "Yes, but I have something he will never have ... *Enough.*"xxxvii

SELF-CARE PRACTICES

Heller understood *enough* and contentment; he was not chasing more and falling into the traps and harmful desires we are warned about in 1 Timothy. His love was not for money; he was not eager for more money, being tempted to make poor decisions just to obtain more wealth. That was the key that unlocked the chains of guilt, shame, and embarrassment for me. When I ask for payment from clients or need to discuss money with my financial advisor, I remind myself that all the money I ask for, receive, and use is a tool that can be used for positive outcomes and to further the kingdom of God. With all of this in mind, here are some things you can do to practice financial wellness.

Set clear goals and intentions for your finances

Take time to write out your financial and career objectives, then create a budget plan to help you stay on track. Journaling your intentions and tracking your progress can be powerful tools for staying motivated and focused. As Proverbs 21:5 reminds us, "The plans of the diligent lead to profit as surely as haste leads to poverty." This verse underscores the value of thoughtful financial planning and intentional money management.

Careful preparation, such as aligning your finances with your priorities, often leads to peace of mind and stability. While even the best plans can encounter unforeseen challenges, the wisdom of planning remains undeniable. Neglecting to plan or set financial intentions often results in unnecessary stress and missed opportunities. Take the time to design your financial journey with purpose; your future self will thank you.

Say NO to peer pressure spending

Along with careful planning, set healthy boundaries for yourself and your finances. You don't have to keep up with everyone else. If friends or family are pressuring you to join in on a big vacation, buy expensive gifts, or dine at a fancy restaurant, and it doesn't align with your financial goals, it's OK to decline politely. Prioritize what matters most to you and your journey toward financial wellness.

Ecclesiastes 4:4 states, "And I saw that all toil and all achievement spring from one person's envy of another. This too is meaningless, a chasing after the wind." This verse reminds us of the futility of comparison and competition. The drive to spend or achieve often stems not from personal desires or needs but from a pressure to measure up to others. Much like chasing the wind, this constant striving leads to frustration and a lack of fulfillment.

Instead of chasing the fleeting approval of others, focus on what brings genuine joy and aligns with your values. True financial wellness isn't about impressing others or keeping up appearances; it's about finding contentment, practicing stewardship, and living within your means in a way that honors your priorities and goals.

Seek wisdom and counsel

Just as Proverbs 15:22 reminds us, "Plans fail for lack of counsel, but with many advisers they succeed." Seeking guidance and wisdom is a powerful step toward financial wellness. Consider hiring a financial coach or certified financial planner to help you navigate your unique financial situation. Take an online course or attend a class at a local college to gain deeper insights into money management, investing, and financial planning.

Learning something new and becoming more informed equips you to make better decisions for the future. Yet, we often put these kinds of opportunities on the back burner, prioritizing immediate needs over long-term growth. Remember that gaining financial knowledge is an act of stewardship—a way to honor God by managing His blessings wisely. I like how Proverbs 4:7 is written in the NLT version, "Getting wisdom is the wisest thing you can do! And whatever else you do, develop good judgment." Investing in your financial education is not just practical; it's a way to align your actions with biblical principles of diligence and wisdom.

Don't hesitate to seek out trustworthy advisers or mentors who can guide you along this path. Their insights, coupled with your dedication to learning, can help you build a strong foundation for a more secure and faithful financial future.

Treat yourself to something nice

There is no sin in spending some of your hard-earned money on yourself. The idea that you must give away everything and live in poverty to honor God is a misconception. Ecclesiastes 3:13 reminds us, "That each of them may eat and drink, and find satisfaction in all their toil—this is the gift of God." God has blessed you with resources not only to share and steward wisely but also to enjoy.

Treating yourself is part of acknowledging and appreciating the blessings in your life. Buying that eight-dollar latte, picking up fresh flowers at the grocery store, or splurging on something small that brings you joy is not only permissible but can be a way to practice gratitude and celebrate the fruits of your labor.

Of course, balance is key. Proverbs 21:20 says, "The wise store up choice food and olive oil, but fools gulp theirs down." While we should use our resources wisely and work toward our goals, finding joy in the journey is equally important. Treating yourself to little luxuries doesn't mean you're failing to manage your finances—it's a way to refresh your spirit and maintain a healthy relationship with money. Enjoy these moments guilt-free, knowing that you're honoring both your hard work and the blessings God has provided.

I want to wrap up this chapter by offering some fresh perspectives and new ways of thinking about money. Financial wellness deserves the same attention and intentionality as every other area of wellness we've discussed in this book. It's time we break the stigma and create space for open, honest conversations about finances. You should never feel embarrassed or ashamed about financial struggles, nor should you feel guilty for having wealth or a solid retirement plan.

The real issue isn't about how much or how little you have; it's about where your heart is and what you are relying on. Matthew 6:21 reminds us, "For where your treasure is, there your heart will be also." Are you trusting God to meet your needs, or are you placing your hope and security in your financial status? The danger lies not in being poor or wealthy but in becoming disconnected from God's purpose for your life.

Money is a tool, a resource to be used wisely, generously, and with gratitude. Let's approach financial wellness with faith, humility, and the understanding that true security and fulfillment come from God alone.

Where do you put your Hope?

> **Timothy 6:17-19**: Command those who are **rich** in this present world not to be *arrogant* nor to put their hope in **wealth**, which is so uncertain, but to put their *hope in God*, who **richly** provides us with everything for *our* enjoyment. Command them to do good, to be **rich** in good deeds, and to be *generous* and *willing to share*. In this way, they will lay up **treasure** for themselves as a firm foundation for the coming age, so that they may take hold of the life that is truly life (emphasis mine).

Conclusion

I hope this book has helped you see the importance and value of self-care and how to put it into practice. Refer back to the end of each chapter to find practical habits and actionable steps to implement self-care strategies in your daily life. The more I study psychology and dive into scripture, the more I see the beautiful blending of science and the Word of God. Whether it's how God provided for Ruth and Naomi in a way that reflects Maslow's hierarchy of needs or how Jesus built trust and connection with His disciples, one truth remains clear: the Bible's timeless truth.

Science often feels like a discovery process, uncovering principles and truths that God has already woven into creation. The more we understand how the mind, body, and soul work together, the more we see that scripture has always been ahead of us, providing a roadmap for a healthy, joyful, and balanced life.

What if we truly lived out the teachings of the Bible? What if we trusted its wisdom, sought its guidance, and allowed it to shape not only our spiritual lives but also our emotional, mental, and physical well-being? I believe we would be healthier, more resilient, and experience a deeper joy that is not dependent on circumstances but rooted in a *peace that surpasses understanding.*

Throughout this book, we've explored self-care through the lens of deep health in seven key areas of wellness. Let's review:

Megan Wollerton

Purpose/Existential

In the Purpose/Existential Wellness chapter, we learned that having a clear sense of purpose, your "reason for being," is essential for living a meaningful and fulfilling life. Drawing inspiration from the Japanese concept of *ikigai*, we explored how aligning what you love, what you're good at, what you can be paid for, and what the world needs can create a life of balance and intention. Studies show that a strong sense of purpose improves mental health, reduces the risk of chronic disease, and builds resilience. Practicing purpose-driven self-care, such as reflecting on your achievements, setting meaningful goals and journaling about them, praying, meditating, and engaging with your faith community can deepen your connection to God's plan and help you live with greater fulfillment. Jeremiah 29:11 reminds us, *God has a plan for each of us, giving us hope and a future when we seek Him with all our hearts.*

Mental

The Mental Wellness chapter taught us that mental health is about cognitive function, clear thinking, problem-solving, memory, and focus. Cognitive flexibility is key to adapting to change, managing stress, and staying resilient. Chronic stress can harm cognitive health, but practices like gratitude journaling, meditation, brain training, and lifelong learning help protect it. Practicing mental wellness and self-care can enhance focus, improve decision-making, and build resilience against life's challenges. Scripture emphasizes wisdom and continuous learning, reminding us that nurturing our minds is both a practical and spiritual responsibility.

Emotional

The Emotional Wellness chapter taught us that emotional wellness involves understanding, managing, and expressing emotions constructively, allowing us to navigate life's highs and lows without getting stuck in any single feeling. Emotional wellness is not about being happy all the time but embracing a wide range of emotions and avoiding toxic positivity. Chronic stress and burnout were explored, along with the physical and emotional impacts of emotional dysregulation. Practical self-care practices such as labeling emotions, talking to a trusted friend or counselor, finding joy, engaging in creativity, and focusing on God's promises help build emotional resilience. Scripture reminds us that while we will face challenges, God's guidance, prayer, and gratitude provide peace and strength to overcome them.

Physical

In the Physical Wellness chapter, we learned that caring for our bodies is an act of gratitude and stewardship for the precious gift God has given us. Physical wellness isn't about perfection or extremes but making small, consistent changes in three key areas: sleep, nutrition, and activity. Sleep restores our minds and bodies, nutrition fuels us with the nourishment we need, and movement keeps us strong and energized. By viewing our bodies as temples of the Holy Spirit, we shift from "I should" to "I want" when it comes to caring for them. Simple practices like creating sleep rituals, eating more fruits and vegetables, and finding ways to move throughout the day can significantly improve our physical and spiritual well-being. As 1 Corinthians 6:19-20 remind us, honoring our bodies is a way to honor God, enabling us to pursue the purposes He has for our lives fully.

Environmental

In the Environmental Wellness chapter, we learned that the spaces we inhabit, both indoors and outdoors, play a crucial role in supporting our physical, mental, and emotional well-being. Environmental wellness involves creating healthy, stimulating surroundings, whether through spending time in nature with activities like forest bathing or intentionally organizing our indoor spaces to promote success and relaxation. Practices like minimizing distractions, setting up environments for better sleep, and even simple activities like gardening can significantly enhance our health. Scripture reminds us that God designed the earth for us to care for and enjoy, and prioritizing our environment is a form of stewardship that honors His creation while promoting our overall wellness.

Relational

In the Relational Wellness chapter, we learned that relationships are foundational to our well-being, impacting our mental, emotional, and even physical health. Humans are designed for connection, as evidenced by both biblical teachings and scientific research. Supportive relationships enhance resilience, reduce stress, and foster personal growth, while isolation can lead to significant health challenges. Building meaningful connections requires intentional effort, such as regular communication, acts of kindness, and spending quality time with loved ones. Scripture reminds us of the power of community, emphasizing that we grow and thrive when surrounded by wise, encouraging, and loving people. Relationships are part of God's design for joy, growth, and purpose, reminding us that we are stronger together than alone.

Financial

In the Financial Wellness chapter, we learned that managing money with confidence and aligning financial decisions with our values reduces stress and improves overall well-being. Financial wellness isn't about how much we have but how we use it as a tool for good, reflecting stewardship, generosity, and trust in God's provision (Matthew 6:21, 1 Timothy 6:17-19). By setting clear goals, resisting peer pressure spending, seeking financial wisdom, and finding joy in our blessings, we honor God and create a healthy relationship with money. True financial wellness comes from balance, gratitude, and placing our hope in God, not wealth.

As you progress in your wellness journey, I encourage you to apply what you've learned in this book. Start small but start intentionally. Seek God first in all things, embrace the truths in His Word, and nurture the life He has given you. When we live as stewards of our health, time, and relationships, we glorify Him while also creating space for His blessings to overflow in our lives.

Remember, you don't have to navigate this journey alone. If you're unsure where to start or how to maintain balance in your life, I invite you to take the **free Life Balance Assessment** at www.burdenedtobalancedbook.com. This quick assessment will help you identify areas that need attention and provide personalized insights to guide your next steps.

If you're ready for deeper transformation, whether for yourself or your organization, I'd love to support you personally. **Book a free call** with me through the website to explore how one-on-one coaching can help you create sustainable habits, overcome burnout, and reclaim balance in your life.

I hope this book has helped you move from feeling burdened to achieving balance. This journey is not just a series of steps; it is a transformation that God invites us to embrace each day. My prayer is that you find renewal, strength, and purpose as you follow this path. Remember, you are not alone. You are loved, and you are equipped to thrive.

> **Matthew 11:28-30**: *Come to me, all you who are weary and burdened, and I will give you rest.* Take my yoke upon you and learn from me, for I am gentle and humble in heart, and you will find rest for your souls. For my yoke is easy and my burden is light (NIV, emphasis mine).
> *The God of peace be with you all. Amen.*

About the Author

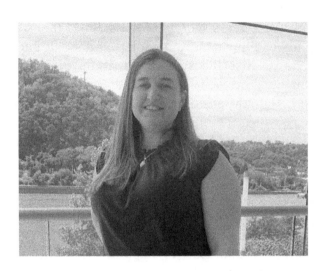

Megan Wollerton
B.S. Business Administration/Marketing, Minor in Psychology - Edinboro University
Certified Personal Trainer, Certified Health Coach, Certified Nutrition Coach, Certified Corporate Wellness Specialist, Certified Positive Psychology Practitioner and Certified Stress Management, Sleep and Recovery Coach.

Megan Wollerton, owner of Life Force Wellness LLC, is a certified personal trainer, health coach, nutrition coach, corporate wellness specialist, and positive psychology practitioner. She is also a stress management, sleep, and recovery coach. With a B.S. in business administration/marketing and a minor in psychology, Megan has a passion for coaching individuals and creating engaging corporate wellness programs that work for both employees and employers.

After experiencing burnout working long, stressful hours in the tumultuous oil and gas field, Megan decided to break out on her own and focus on health and wellness. She recognized the importance of work-life balance and created a program that would benefit herself and her employees. Since then, Megan has been helping clients achieve happier and healthier lifestyles through her expertise in exercise, nutrition, mental resiliency, behavior change, and well-being. Megan brings her passion for wellness into the corporate environment by collaborating with leaders to transform company cultures, emphasizing employee health and wellbeing. Her mission is to create psychologically safe and less toxic working environments where employees can thrive.

At Life Force Wellness, Megan focuses on seven distinct areas of well-being. With her dedication to helping others and extensive knowledge of wellness, she is committed to providing effective solutions that lead to happier and more productive employees for companies.

Works Cited

---

[i] HR. "Brené Brown About Fitting in and True Belonging #Shorts," June 14, 2023, https://www.youtube.com/watch?v=2ClCPF9w7yc.

[ii] Precision Nutrition, "Precision Nutrition Level 1 Nutrition Coaching Certification."

[iii] Okuzono, Sakurako S et al. "Ikigai and subsequent health and wellbeing among Japanese older adults: Longitudinal outcome-wide analysis." *The Lancet regional health. Western Pacific* vol. 21 100391. 3 Feb. 2022, doi: 10.1016/j.lanwpc.2022.100391, https://pmc.ncbi.nlm.nih.gov/articles/PMC8814687/.

[iv] Sone T, Nakaya N, Ohmori K, Shimazu T, Higashiguchi M, Kakizaki M, Kikuchi N, Kuriyama S, Tsuji I. Sense of life worth living (ikigai) and mortality in Japan: Ohsaki Study. Psychosom Med. 2008 Jul;70(6):709-15. doi: 10.1097/PSY.0b013e31817e7e64. Epub 2008 Jul 2. PMID: 18596247, https://pubmed.ncbi.nlm.nih.gov/18596247/

[v] Shraddha A. Shende, Raksha A. Mudar, Cognitive control in age-related hearing loss: A narrative review, Hearing Research, Vol. 436, 2023, 108814, ISSN 0378-5955, https://www.sciencedirect.com/topics/neuroscience/cognitive-flexibility

[vi] Justin Trudeau, "Justine Trudeau's Davos address in Full," World Economic Forum, (January 23, 2018), https://www.weforum.org/stories/2018/01/pm-keynote-remarks-for-world-economic-forum-2018/.

[vii] Find more information here: https://www.nia.nih.gov/health/brain-health/cognitive-health-and-older-adults or here https://pmc.ncbi.nlm.nih.gov/articles/PMC3934012/

viii Hutton JS, Dudley J, Horowitz-Kraus T, DeWitt T, Holland SK. Associations Between Screen-Based Media Use and Brain White Matter Integrity in Preschool-Aged Children. *JAMA Pediatr.* 2020;174(1):e193869. doi:10.1001/jamapediatrics.2019.3869

ix JAMA Pediatr. 2020 Jan 1;174(1):e193869. doi: 10.1001/jamapediatrics.2019.3869. Epub 2020 Jan 6.

x https://www.azquotes.com/quote/486048

xi Schultz SA, Larson J, Oh J, Koscik R, Dowling MN, Gallagher CL, Carlsson CM, Rowley HA, Bendlin BB, Asthana S, Hermann BP, Johnson SC, Sager M, LaRue A, Okonkwo OC. Participation in cognitively-stimulating activities is associated with brain structure and cognitive function in preclinical Alzheimer's disease. Brain Imaging Behav. 2015 Dec;9(4):729-36. doi: 10.1007/s11682-014-9329-5. PMID: 25358750; PMCID: PMC4417099.

xii Weaver AN, Jaeggi SM. Activity Engagement and Cognitive Performance Amongst Older Adults. Front Psychol. 2021 Mar 11;12:620867. doi: 10.3389/fpsyg.2021.620867. PMID: 33776844; PMCID: PMC7990770.

xiii Radostina K. Purvanova, John P. Muros, "Gender differences in burnout: A meta-analysis," *Journal of Vocational Behavior* 77, no. 2 (2010): 168-185, https://www.sciencedirect.com/science/article/abs/pii/S0001879110000771.

xiv Nicole M. Caulfield, Aleksandr T. Karnick, Daniel W. Capron, "Exploring dissociation as a facilitator of suicide risk: A translational investigation using virtual reality," *Journal of Affective Disorders* 297, (2022): 517-524, https://www.sciencedirect.com/science/article/pii/S0165032721011885.

xv American Psychological Association, "Stress in America 2023: A nation recovering from collective trauma," November 2023, https://www.apa.org/news/press/releases/stress/2023/collective-trauma-recovery#:~:text=Most%20cited%20anxiety%20disorder%20(24%)%2 oor%20depression,because%20they%20know%20others%20have%20it%20worse.

xvi John Bevere, "A Spirit of Fear Versus Fear of the Lord," Bible Gateway Blog, February 20, 2023, https://www.biblegateway.com/blog/2023/02/a-spirit-of-fear-versus-fear-of-the-lord/.

xvii Gavin de Becker, *The Gift of Fear*, (New York: Dell Publishing, a division of Random House, Inc., 1997).

xviii Bible Gateway, https://www.biblegateway.com/resources/encyclopedia-of-the-bible/Joy.

xix Quotes.net, STANDS4 LLC, 2025. "Bambi Quotes." Accessed March 6, 2025, https://www.quotes.net/movies/bambi_quotes_736.

xx National Center for Chronic Disease Prevention and Health Promotion (NCCDPHP), "What You Can Do to Meet Physical Activity Recommendations, April 16, 2024, https://www.cdc.gov/physical-activity-basics/guidelines/index.html.

xxi National Center for Chronic Disease Prevention and Health Promotion (NCCDPHP), "What You Can Do to Meet Physical Activity Recommendations, April 16, 2024, https://www.cdc.gov/physical-activity-basics/guidelines/index.html.

xxii https://www.cdc.gov/physical-activity-basics/guidelines/index.html

xxiii Susan Linney, "What is HALT? The Dangers of Being Hungry, Angry, Lonely or Tired," American Addiction Centers, January 5, 2024, https://americanaddictioncenters.org/blog/common-stressors-recovery.

xxiv https://www.nationalgeographic.com/travel/article/forest-bathing-nature-walk-health#:~:text=The%20term%20emerged%20in%20Japan%20in%20the,reconnect%20with%20and%20protect%20the%20country's%20forests xxv White, M.P., Alcock, I., Grellier, J. et al. "Spending at least 120 minutes a week in nature is associated with good health and wellbeing." *Sci Rep* 9, 7730 (2019), https://doi.org/10.1038/s41598-019-44097-3, https://rdcu.be/ecDKL.

xxvi https://ntrs.nasa.gov/citations/19930073077

xxvii https://pmc.ncbi.nlm.nih.gov/articles/PMC4449931/#:~:text=(Peart%201992).-,Chlorophytum%20comosum%20L.,Peart%201992;%20Giese%20et%20al.

xxviii Richard Weissbourd, Milena Batanova, Virginia Lovison, and Eric Torres, "Loneliness in America: How the Pandemic Has Deepened an Epidemic of Loneliness and What We Can Do About It," Harvard Graduate School of Education, (February 2021), https://mcc.gse.harvard.edu/reports/loneliness-in-america.

xxix https://www.sciencedirect.com/topics/medicine-and-dentistry/triune-brain#:~:text=To%20understand%20unconscious%20components%2C%20the,processing%20assembly%E2%80%9D%20at%20each%20stage.

xxx Saul McLeod, PhD, "Maslow's Hierarchy of Needs," *Simply Psychology*, (January 24, 2024), https://www.simplypsychology.org/maslow.html#:~:text=According%20to%20Maslow%20(1943%2C%201954,can%20satisfy%20the%20higher%20needs.

xxxi Eisenberger, Naomi I et al. "Does rejection hurt? An FMRI study of social exclusion." *Science (New York, N.Y.)* vol. 302,5643 (2003): 290-2. doi:10.1126/science.1089134, https://pubmed.ncbi.nlm.nih.gov/14551436/.

xxxii Alotaibi, Turki A et al. "The Benefits of Friendships in Academic Settings: A Systematic Review and Meta-Analysis." *Cureus* vol. 15,12 e50946. 22 Dec. 2023, doi:10.7759/cureus.50946, https://pmc.ncbi.nlm.nih.gov/articles/PMC10800095/.

xxxiii PwC, "PwC's 2023 Employee Financial Wellness Survey: Guiding your employees through uncertain economic times," https://www.pwc.com/us/en/services/consulting/business-transformation/library/employee-financial-wellness-survey.html.

xxxiv
https://pmc.ncbi.nlm.nih.gov/articles/PMC8806009/#:~:text=Psychological%20distress%20was%20measured%20using,the%20lack%20of%20coping%20resources.

https://www.purdue.edu/newsroom/archive/purduetoday/releases/2021/Q1/mental-well-being-inherently-connected-to-financial-wellness.html#:~:text=The%20link%20between%20mental%20health%20and%20financial,are%20more%20connected%20than%20some%20may%20realize.&text=High%20levels%20of%20financial%20stress%2C%20as%20with,depression%20and%20a%20feeling%20of%20being%20overwhelmed.

xxxv Bible Gateway,
https://www.biblegateway.com/quicksearch/?quicksearch=wealth&version=NIV.
https://www.biblegateway.com/quicksearch/?quicksearch=money&version=NIV
https://www.biblegateway.com/quicksearch/?quicksearch=money&version=NIV
https://www.biblegateway.com/quicksearch/?quicksearch=shekels&version=NIV

xxxvi P.T. Barnum, *The Art of Money Getting: Golden Rules for Making Money*, "The Art of Money Getting Quotes," Goodreads, https://www.goodreads.com/work/quotes/1404893-the-art-of-money-getting-or-golden-rules-for-making-money

xxxvii John C. Bogle, "Enough,"
https://www.johncbogle.com/wordpress/wp-content/uploads/2007/05/Georgetown_2007.pdf

www.ingramcontent.com/pod-product-compliance
Lightning Source LLC
LaVergne TN
LVHW022002040425
807748LV00008B/354